five lessons
I didn't
learn from
breast cancer

(and One Big One I Did)

five lessons
I didn't
learn from
breast cancer

(and One Big One I Did)

Shelley Lewis

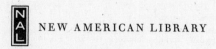
NEW AMERICAN LIBRARY

New American Library
Published by New American Library, a division of Penguin Group (USA) Inc., 375 Hudson
Street, New York, New York 10014, USA • Penguin Group (Canada), 90 Eglinton Avenue
East, Suite 700, Toronto, Ontario M4P 2Y3, Canada (a division of Pearson Penguin Can-
ada Inc.) • Penguin Books Ltd., 80 Strand, London WC2R 0RL, England • Penguin
Ireland, 25 St. Stephen's Green, Dublin 2, Ireland (a division of Penguin Books Ltd.) •
Penguin Group (Australia), 250 Camberwell Road, Camberwell, Victoria 3124, Australia
(a division of Pearson Australia Group Pty. Ltd.) • Penguin Books India Pvt. Ltd., 11
Community Centre, Panchsheel Park, New Delhi - 110 017, India • Penguin Group (NZ),
67 Apollo Drive, Rosedale, North Shore 0632, New Zealand (a division of Pearson New
Zealand Ltd.) • Penguin Books (South Africa) (Pty.) Ltd., 24 Sturdee Avenue, Rosebank,
Johannesburg 2196, South Africa

Penguin Books Ltd., Registered Offices:
80 Strand, London WC2R 0RL, England

First published by New American Library,
a division of Penguin Group (USA) Inc.

First Printing, May 2008
10 9 8 7 6 5 4 3 2 1

REGISTERED TRADEMARK—MARCA REGISTRADA

LIBRARY OF CONGRESS CATALOGING-IN-PUBLICATION DATA
Lewis, Shelley.
    Five lessons I didn't learn from breast cancer (and one big one I did)/Shelley Lewis.
      p. cm.
    ISBN 978-0-451-22390-6
    1. Lewis, Shelley—Health.   2. Breast—Cancer—Patient—Biography.   I. Title.
RC280.B8L383 2008
362.196' 994490092—dc22   2007049705

Set in Walbaum MT with ITC Syndor   •   Designed by Sabrina Bowers

Printed in the United States of America

PUBLISHER'S NOTE
While the author has made every effort to provide accurate telephone numbers and Internet
addresses at the time of publication, neither the publisher nor the author assumes any
responsibility for errors, or for changes that occur after publication. Further, publisher
does not have any control over and does not assume any responsibility for author or
third-party Web sites or their content.

Contents

Contents

PART 3:
The After (Cancer) Life

Acknowledgments

I am very grateful that I didn't have to go through this difficult journey alone. There were many dark times when my spirits flagged, and I just wasn't sure I could get to the finish line. Luckily I had many friends and professionals to provide the emotional and intellectual support I needed.

Writing a book is so hard.

Oh, wait, you thought I was talking about breast cancer, didn't you? I'll get to that, but first things first.

I want to thank all of the women who contributed their stories, their insights, and their time so generously to this book. They allowed me to create a fuller picture of what the modern breast cancer experience actually is for many women. Dr. Bonni Gearhart was my medical consultant on the book, and her help was invaluable. She's also a delightful, funny, smart chick whose patients adore her. Thanks to my business partner and friend, Joanna Breen, who listened, and waited (relatively) patiently when I had to juggle our work with the writing of this book. And I was so fortunate to have the advice and counsel of my wise and talented editor, Tracy Bernstein, who laughed at my jokes even when she'd read them four times. My dear friend, who is also my agent, Laurie Liss, encouraged me to write about my breast cancer adventure after going through much of it with me.

Now, about that breast cancer thing: I had an abundance of love and support with that too, starting with my husband, Dennis Kardon and my daughter, Julia Kardon. Enormous thanks also to: my friend Rachel Bellow, who held my hand through chemo and made me laugh; my sister, Lisa Lewis, who was my go-to person when research needed to be done; my Air America colleagues, Jon Sinton in particular, whose kindnesses began on day one. And of course, I thank my doctors, who were unfailingly thoughtful, careful and collaborative, and best of all, successful, at least so far.

I am blessed with wonderful parents—a mother whom I can always count on to be my most enthusiastic cheerleader, and a father whose influence on who I am can't be overstated. So most of all I thank my dad, Leonard Lewis, who has always made me feel I was the smartest girl in the room, and that I (usually) have something interesting to say. I am very proud to be his daughter.

five lessons
I didn't
learn from
breast cancer

(and One Big One I Did)

Introduction

"Life is what happens to you when you're busy making other plans."

—*John Lennon*

Experts say that when faced with a personal crisis, every human will go through at least two of the five stages of grief (denial, anger, bargaining, depression, and acceptance). When I discovered I had breast cancer, I was no exception:

Dear God: WTF???

Are you freaking kidding me? This has got to be some huge mistake.

No?

Really?

But why me, God? What did I do to deserve this?

Was it my diet?

My exercise regimen?

The fact that I didn't have one?

Did I do something morally reprehensible just when You happened to be watching?

Hey, if I'm being punished, there are plenty of other people who deserve it more than I do. And I'm willing to name names.

Wait, I got it. You can just undo this. You're God, after all.

Well, if You think I'm going to be transformed into a better person, forget it. You just wasted a perfectly good case of early-stage breast cancer on me.

Oh, and thanks for totally screwing up my summer.

I guess you could say my relationship with God has been problematic for both of us.

Okay, you know the one-sided conversation above is a joke, right? I didn't *really* believe I knew plenty of people who deserved it, any more than I did, and although I had a lot of questions when I found out I had breast cancer (like "Are you sure?"), "Why me?" wasn't one of them. I didn't ask God anything, except maybe once when I was praying not to get dry heaves after someone came into a meeting with a container of Thai food.

There's no more to be gained from pondering why you were chosen to get breast cancer than there is from wondering why you were chosen to have an overbite, or facial hair, or an extra toe.

Unless you have the BRCA gene mutation that places you at much higher risk to develop breast cancer, the odds are you'll never know why you, of all people, got it. What the medical community really knows for sure about the causes of breast cancer could be printed on the back of a pink ribbon and still leave room for a coupon to buy a "huggable" stuffed animal from the Breast Cancer Mall. Let's agree that we aren't going to waste any time on questions that can't be answered and focus on the ones that can be.

The first question isn't "Why do I have this problem?"; it's "How do I solve this problem?"

And the answer is, you'll solve it the way you solve all of the challenges you confront. You bring a lifetime of experience, skills, and wisdom to breast cancer. We all do.

Cancer didn't teach me lessons that changed my life; my life taught me lessons that changed my cancer experience. Hence, the title of this book.

Not that my turn in Breast Cancer Club was all smooth sailing, or a nice, calm experience, beginning to end. There were plenty of quiet freak-outs.

But I do think I was mostly able to keep the panic attacks at bay by being as prepared as possible for the various terrifying situations I faced.

I'm no expert, but I'll tell you everything I know. And better still, I've included the good advice contributed by the many wise and strong women I've met while writing this book. I've learned from all of them. You will, too.

I can promise you, there will be no brave laughing through the tears, no tales of my heroic struggles.

For one thing, I'm not brave. I'm kind of a coward, especially around needles. And I'm definitely not a hero. A hero is someone who does something brave and noble because it's the right thing to do, not because she has no choice. I just did what I was told, more or less.

Breast cancer wasn't a journey that led me to anywhere worth going, and you will never, ever hear me say I was glad I had it, for any reason. It's true that because of breast cancer I have met some wonderful and lovely women who have enriched my life, but while having coffee with two of them recently, we all agreed that if given the choice between having breast cancer or having one another for friends, we'd rather not have met at all. And sure, we learned some stuff, but all things considered, we'd rather just take a course from one of those online colleges, or go to the Learning Annex.

This is not a book filled with "look on the bright side" advice.

This is a book for women who don't have and don't want a spiritual makeover after breast cancer. We like who we are, and we like our lives. And we don't expect cancer to fix what's wrong with them.

I was surprised to find that a life-threatening experience did not become a life-altering one. But now I realize it's completely life-affirming to want to remain who you essentially are, good traits and bad, rather than make permanent accommodations for a disease that you have to believe is just passing through.

I came out on the other side of breast cancer pretty much the same person I was going into it.

My only growth was the one removed by my surgeon.

This book features many other women who share that view. We refused to be pink-wrapped, infantilized, put on a pedestal or put on the sidelines. We aren't looking for a karmic reward for going through cancer—survival is its own reward.

And we don't think we deserve a spiritual rebirth, any more than we deserved to get breast cancer.

That's not to say I didn't learn things about myself from the experience; of course I did. For one thing, I learned how clueless I was about breast cancer, when it was unwrapped from the soft pink packaging that had lulled me into thinking, *Well, okay, even if you do get it, it won't be that bad. It's so curable these days.*

When I had breast cancer, everybody I told responded by telling me about someone else she knew who'd had breast cancer, too. I knew that was supposed to give me confidence, but it didn't, really. A little voice in my head was whispering, "Yes, but..." Finally, when my friend Rachel said to me, "You're not scared, are you? I mean, I know so many women who've had it and then they're just fine," I was surprised to hear myself practically shout, "Yes, but this time it's *me*."

Since you're reading this, odds are this time it's you. Or it was you.

You will get through this. It will suck at times, for sure, but it will not be more than you can handle. Here's a little secret:

You don't have to have a TV movie version of your breast cancer. You don't have to have the experience you've read about a million times in women's magazines and *People*.

Lots of us decide we don't have to stop our lives to have cancer with all the trimmings—support groups, chat room visits, survivor walks. You don't see a lot of television or magazine stories about those of us trying to keep breast cancer's impact to a minimum. (It doesn't make for great television, for one thing.) But we're there.

I realized fairly quickly that I didn't want to do any of the things I thought were expected of me. I didn't want to go to a support group, either to support or to be supported. I was too fragile then.

I was spooked by the very thought of sitting in a chemo room knitting and sharing my chemo emo with the patient in the next chair. When I'd had my treatment I escaped that room as quickly as I could. I wanted to flee the land of the sick so I could run back to the place I believed I belonged, which was the world of the thoughtlessly, carelessly healthy.

I felt about Cancer Club the same way I did when I got my first invitation to join AARP.

Yikes, no way am I doing this. Throw that thing out before someone sees you with it.

Cancer Club is a perverse organization where you pay your dues in order to be let out, not in. But even if you throw out the membership card, once they send it to you, you're in it.

AARP is only slightly less persistent.

I do not have an AARP card—I just can't do it—and I only show my Cancer Card on select occasions (more about that later), but I do not accept all the customs that many club members seem to enjoy.

Like, I draw the line at "Cancer was a gift." You read it and hear it a lot around the clubhouse.

Why that has wormed its way into the received wisdom about cancer I do not know, but I think I will blame it on celebrities, because there are numerous examples of famous people who've said their cancer was a gift, or that it made them a better person. I won't name any names, but one of them rhymes with Pants Sharmstrong.

It just may be that you won't have an epiphany about the meaning of life, either. And you may not think of cancer as your ultimate self-improvement opportunity. If that's the case, you can join our chapter of the club. We're working on a cool Latin motto, maybe changing the old "In vino veritas," which means "In wine, there is truth"—something every woman who has ever drunk-dialed an ex-boyfriend understands—to "In chemo veritas." Either that or "*Stercus accidit*," which I'm told means "Shit happens."

For at least a year after I had breast cancer, my friends would ask me what I'd learned from it. And I admit I fell prey to the media hype a little. I did think there ought to be something I could point to. I mean, I hated to let everybody down. You should have seen me, trying to find some pearl of wisdom when my friends asked me how breast cancer had changed me. But I had nothing. Nada.

I Went on a Spiritual Cancer Journey and All I Brought Back Was This Lousy Attitude.

I think the closest I ever came to a major change in my philosophy of life was when I announced I was going to give up Botox (and really, that was because I didn't like the way it made my eyebrows arch like Agnes Moorehead's in *Bewitched*).

I did wonder sometimes if I had some kind of character flaw. It didn't bother me much but I was kind of curious—was I now officially the shallowest woman on the planet? And if so, is there a reality show in my future?

Finally, I was at a party, talking with an acquaintance who'd had breast cancer the year before I did. I confessed to her that try as I might, I couldn't point to a single way in which cancer had improved me as a person.

She chuckled and said, "Me neither. Stop trying. Haven't you done enough? You made it."

She was absolutely right.

Breast cancer didn't change who I was; it confirmed who I was. What was important to me before was still important to me after. My core values not only didn't change because of breast cancer, they are what got me through it. I am who I am, I am who I always was (give or take a divot in my right breast).

I found my own higher power by digging deeper into myself. Everything I've learned, all the places I've been, my successes and failures, were available to me there, and they were the survival guide I needed.

If you're going through treatment, know that you can access your own incredible reserves of wisdom and common sense and strength. Hell, if I can do it, you can do it.

Sometimes I wish I *had* benefited, the way others apparently have, from breast cancer. It would be great to have become more spiritual, a kinder, gentler soul, or to have achieved a bit of grace about life and the nasty curveballs it throws us. But those are goals I've had for myself practically forever. If I achieve them, am I really supposed to give the credit to a disease? That would give breast cancer the last word. And I'm just not gonna do that.

I've spent a lifetime getting myself into and out of jams, some of them self-created, some, like breast cancer, totally not my fault. I believe that it's important to learn from your mistakes, but it's even better when you can learn from somebody else's, so the Five Lessons include a lot of what not to do, as contributed by some of the smart, funny, strong women who participated so generously in this book.

From the truth about lying to yourself (it's sooo helpful), to sex and the single (breasted) girl, to acknowledging that it's your kids' world and you're just barfing in it, to whether we really need a ribbon for Acid Reflux Awareness (I'm not kidding), to why Pink Ribbon Barbie should be stripped, head shaved, and forced to replace her pink tulle dress with a green hospital gown, I think you'll find plenty of useful observations here.

So let's begin with the importance of being shallow.

Part One

*STERCUS ACCIDIT**

*Sh*t happens

Chapter One

Take Human Bites

```
┌─────────────────────────────────────┐
│  Lesson One:                        │
│  Denial is your new best friend.    │
│  Embrace it. Make it work for       │
│  you. Do not give it nights or      │
│  weekends off.                      │
└─────────────────────────────────────┘
```

"Being on the tightrope is living; everything else is waiting."

—Karl Wallenda, world-famous tightrope walker

Life, Without a Net

Not a lot of people get their career advice from Karl Wallenda, and, in hindsight, I can see why. You'd better have a finely developed sense of denial to get up for tightrope walking every day. You'd need a voice in your head saying, "You can do this! What could possibly go wrong? Nothing you can't handle, baby." It's kind of like getting yourself psyched up for breast cancer treatment.

It's also like being a television producer, which was what I was for much of my career. Most producers have the professional life spans of a fruit fly, but every time we take on a show, we believe we're going to be wildly successful, despite the odds against us. Maybe there's a little Wallenda in all of us.

I had designated 2004 to be my Year on the Tightrope. I quit my job as executive producer of CNN's *American Morning*, and walked away from more than twenty-five years as a broadcast journalist in what is now known as the mainstream media, to take a chance that the nation's highly charged political climate would support a liberal talk-radio network. Air America Radio, sketched out on a napkin in an Atlanta bar a month before the invasion of Iraq in 2003, seemed to be a risk worth taking.

And, like the Flying Wallendas, I would do my act without a net. If we failed, at least we'd fail huge. In my experience, people will forgive you for taking a flying leap and landing flat on your face. It's not failure that paralyzes you; it's the fear of failure. I have had my share of successes and screwups, and I was not afraid of the challenge.

We were underfinanced and overwhelmed, but somehow we got on the air on March 31, 2004. We had many rough moments those first weeks, but, by God, we had done it. Or so we thought.

One thing we had not done, it turned out, was pay our bills. And that was because money we believed was in the bank in fact was not, for reasons not worth going into here. Air America had almost no money, and nearly all of us missed a paycheck temporarily.

And yet, everybody continued to come to work. We were all in denial; we refused to believe that the network could possibly go under. Every day our new boss would walk by my office and exclaim, "You're here!" and every day I would reply, "Where the hell else would I be?"

Denial gets a bad rap; it can be a very productive mental game if you know when to play it and when to stop. And denial, on a massive group level, is what got us through that crisis at Air America. That, and a few million dollars kicked in at the eleventh hour by some new investors.

So you see, I was already deeply entrenched in the United States of Denial when, just a few weeks after the financial crisis hit, I learned I had breast cancer. Luckily, it's a lot easier to treat breast cancer than it is a seventy-five-foot fall from a tightrope, which put me way ahead of poor Karl Wallenda, who fell off a high wire to his death in 1978.

The Disease I Knew I Would Never Get

In June 2004, I walked into a modern, well-regarded radiology practice on Manhattan's East Side for my annual mammogram. I had been going there for more than ten years, and I liked the fact that you got results from your doctor immediately, on the spot (give or take twenty minutes sitting around in a flimsy gown).

As I entered the reception area I passed a middle-aged

woman whose shiny head was covered with fuzz, like a newborn chick. Clearly, it was regrowth following chemo. That will never be me, I said to myself confidently. Maybe I'll develop cancer someday, but it won't be breast cancer. I believed this because I thought that if there was no breast cancer among your first-degree relatives (defined, in cancer terms, as parent, sibling, or child), you probably wouldn't get it, either. And because I was so sure of that, I didn't find the annual mammogram particularly nerve-racking.

Several times over the years I'd been sent to the sonogram room after my mammogram, to confirm that a dark, scary-looking area in one breast or the other was just a harmless cyst; they always were and they went away on their own. And so it was on that day in June—another probable cyst was discovered, requiring a look-see on the sonogram. No problem. I wasn't at all nervous as I went downstairs to the sonogram suite.

An hour later, after hearing, "Uh-oh, I don't like the looks of that," I was undergoing a core needle biopsy. The doctor who had muttered that unsettling phrase was scooping out bits of breast tissue with a kind of spring-loaded needle. While checking out the cyst (and it *was* just a cyst) she'd detected what she'd called micro-calcifications, which are often the debris left behind by rapidly growing tumor cells, sort of like punks tossing beer cans out the car window as they careen down the highway. The radiologist was very kind, but not optimistic.

Two days later, she called with the results. Just seeing the name of the diagnostic radiology practice on my phone's caller ID screen made my heart pound, but I tried to stay calm as I picked up the receiver and grabbed a notepad and pen. I concentrated as best I could, considering that her voice was competing with the one in my head that was screaming, "Oh, my God . . . are you hearing this? This *cannot* be happening."

Luckily, I'm pretty good at tuning out my hysterical alter ego when she's shrieking in my head. I've had a lot of practice at it.

Concentrating on the doctor's voice, I wrote down words that had little or no meaning to me. As usual, my office door was open, and one of the Air America hosts, Katherine Lanpher, walked in. She took one look at my face and stopped in her tracks. She was perfectly positioned, however, to read over my shoulder, and therefore became the very first person I knew (besides me) to find out I had breast cancer. After she saw the key words, she discreetly withdrew, returning later to offer help. I couldn't imagine what anybody who wasn't wielding a scalpel or a giant vat of valium could do for me at that moment.

As I read over my notes, I focused on a few key things. The tumor was small, it was early, I was lucky. My gynecologist called next, and she described it as "a nice, early catch." I wrote that phrase down and repeated it to everybody I told. Well, sort of told. The fact is I literally couldn't say the words "I have breast cancer." I would mumble something about my situation, and they would invariably be forced to state the obvious. This was rather awkward. As I recall, it went something like this:

> ME: *"So, um, I found out today I have to have a lumpectomy."*
> THEM: *"Wow. Lumpectomy. So you have breast cancer?"*
> ME: *"I don't know. I guess so...apparently. Yeah. I mean, my doctor says it was a nice, early catch."*

I wasn't embarrassed or ashamed of the words "breast cancer." I simply didn't believe it yet. It seemed to be happening to someone else.

Cancer for Twenty Minutes—Let the Denial Begin

And thus began the denial phase, which was my little lifeboat through those first stormy seas. Now, denial takes different forms, but in the case of breast cancer, I think it usually begins with, "There must be some mistake."

Pretty much everybody goes through that, and it's an extremely effective way to stall for time while your brain processes the news. But I was able to add another layer to denial, the "Well, if I *do* have it, it won't be so bad" lie.

If I really did have breast cancer, I told myself, I would have it for like twenty minutes, and then it would be over.

There'd be a lumpectomy, and then some radiation, and ta-dah, done. I also seized on the idea that I would probably be able to lose that five extra pounds I'd been lugging around since winter. (I know, I know, it takes a true optimist or a deeply neurotic person to see a weight-loss opportunity in a cancer diagnosis. I vote for optimist.) In retrospect, I guess I was kind of an idiot. But the media are full of images that say, "Don't worry, you'll be fine"; the plucky, never-say-die Racers for the Cure, the Pink Army of recovered women warriors, young, old, and middle-aged. Isn't that the whole point of the Breast Cancer Awareness campaign, to convince women that it's not such a big deal, at least if you catch it early in your annual mammogram? Well, I was convinced.

Or maybe it was just the lie I told myself because it was what I needed to stay calm and rational. It worked pretty well. It wasn't until a week later, when I first met with my surgeon, Dr. Rache Simmons, that reality smacked me in the face.

You see, my twenty-minute cancer was not supposed to include chemotherapy. After all, I had—wait for it—"a nice, early catch," so why would I need chemo? But Dr. Simmons informed me that in fact it was very likely I would need to have it. I remember gasping when she said it, and that she looked surprised by my reaction.

So much for "it won't be that bad."

It *was* going to be that bad.

If that sounds like I was finally accepting my situation and leaving denial behind, well, not exactly. In fact, here's a confession that I've never even admitted to myself before: While I publicly accepted that I was going to have surgery and probably chemo and radiation, there was a tiny part of me that still wasn't convinced that I really, truly, definitely did have breast cancer. Even after Dr. Simmons showed me the tumor on the mammogram film, I harbored private doubts.

Yeah, okay, I see the little white spot, but what if that's some other woman's breast? I mean, it's just a breast on an X-ray film. Who knows who it belongs to? It could be anybody's.

I think my skepticism was due to the fact that it was impossible to feel the tumor, not just for me but for most of the doctors, too, even when they knew exactly where it was. (For the record, it was at seven o'clock—they actually locate a tumor on a breast by describing its position as if your breast were a clock. Of course, it's from their point of view, not yours. To me, it was five o'clock. Happy Hour.) Anyway, for a long time I secretly suspected it was all some huge mistake, that I was in the wrong place, as if I had walked onto the wrong plane and the doors had closed before I could get off.

But everybody I trusted told me that, in fact, my ticket was stamped for Tumortown, and I was exactly where I was supposed to be. Rationally I had to accept that they were right and I was wrong. I would never, ever have delayed starting treatment; I may have been a little crazy, but I wasn't foolish. And yet . . .

Denial was still my security blanket, and even though

I was being told I had to be a big girl and give it up, I couldn't quite let it go. I was like those kids who carry little corners of their abandoned security blankets in their pockets, so they can secretly finger the threadbare fabric when they want to, without anybody seeing them. It was just weirdly comforting. Denial is a great stalling technique, and who hasn't found herself in a jam where she needed to play for time while she figured out what to do next?

Jessica Stedman Guff was a senior broadcast producer at *Good Morning America*, responsible for all of the stories in the second hour of the show each day. In October of 2006, after producing a segment on breast cancer, she decided to do a self-exam. Sure enough, she found a lump, and although she quickly had it checked out, she wasn't too worried about it. There was no history of breast cancer among her immediate relatives. Even when she was told that her biopsy revealed "abnormal cells," she didn't think that meant she had breast cancer.

"My doctor had to tell me explicitly that my abnormal cells meant I had cancer," she said and chuckled, shaking her head as we talked about it. "I should have known that, but I was too far into denial."

Once Jessica was able to come to terms with her diagnosis, she got to work. Her training as a producer, and as a mother of two kids, kicked in and she did the information gathering and comparison shopping needed to choose a treatment path.

The most important thing to remember about denial is that you can't bask in it forever. It's like a warm bubble bath on a cold morning; eventually you'll have to get out of it if you're going to accomplish anything.

On the other hand, why hurry?

The actress Maria Friedman discovered she had breast cancer ten days before she was scheduled to make her Broadway debut in the musical *The Woman in White.*

"There seemed to be very little point in sort of allowing it to overwhelm me," she said at the time. Five days after a lumpectomy to remove a marble-sized tumor, she was back to rehearsals. A week later, still bruised and bandaged up, with a doctor standing in the wings just in case, she made her Broadway debut in a role that required running, dancing, even fighting, as well as singing. Her bandages were so tight she was having trouble breathing, so her doctor rebandaged her during intermission.

Maria Friedman got to fulfill her dream to open on Broadway by refusing to accept how breast cancer treatment would upset her life. How great was that?

I guess it wasn't too different from me saying, "It won't be that bad." You have to accept your diagnosis, and begin to think about what the process of getting treatment will require of you, but you don't have to anticipate all kinds of ugliness that may or may not come to pass.

Now, denial is kind of an art form. It's not enough just

to stick your fingers in your ears and go "la la la la" real loudly to drown out bad news. You have to convince yourself and the people around you that you are aware of your potentially dire situation, even if, like me, you're secretly not quite there yet.

There are ways to hold on to that soft little scrap of denial in your pocket. One way is to avoid allowing other people to overwhelm you with too much information and unsolicited advice. You deny those people access to your fragile psyche so they can't fill you with their fear.

Another key tactic is to filter the facts. You don't have to take in everything that may happen to you. Not yet. Maybe not ever. You *do* need to accept the first thing, which is that you will have to figure out who will provide your medical care. But the rest you take in bit by bit, as you can handle it.

Taking Human Bites

One of the operating principles of my life is that the world is filled with wisdom and inspiration, if you just take the time to stop and listen. I've learned important lessons from the unlikeliest places.

Like, say, a television commercial from the 1970s that contained these three memorable words:

"Take human bites."

Anyone who lived in New York in the late 1970s probably remembers that ad. It was for a play called *Gemini*, which featured a woman yelling "Take human bites" to her hulking son at the dinner table. It was one of those phrases that everybody used at the time, and not just when they were referring to food. Over the years it has come to represent my idea of great advice for almost any huge problem you have to tackle, including breast cancer. Don't try to digest your diagnosis and your treatment options all in one gulp. It's too overwhelming.

Connecticut governor Jodi Rell, who discovered she had breast cancer just months after taking office, decided to attack her breast cancer as if it were a kind of project.

"When I first found out I had breast cancer, I said, 'You've got to be kidding! I'm the one who promotes awareness—how could this happen to *me*?' " she told me. "But you have to live, you have to keep moving forward. I told myself, 'This is just something you have to deal with now, so just do it. You've got this issue to work through.' I'm methodical, I do things step by step, and I keep going."

In other words, she took human bites. She stayed true to her own way of dealing with a problem, and it worked for her.

The human bite I took was to control the flow of news in and out. The flow in was easy to control; I wrenched myself away from the Internet when I'd had enough. The flow out involved withholding my news from some of my immediate family for a few days. The embargo was meant to keep my not-young parents and not-old daughter from freaking out, and by extension, upsetting me. I hated to keep them in the dark, but I knew that if I told them I had breast cancer when I first found out about it, they would flood me with a tidal wave of questions I couldn't answer, creating more anxiety for all of us. I wanted to spare them and myself that level of upset. So rather than tell them what amounted to a headline, with no details that could allay their fears, I decided to hold back until I'd chosen a surgeon and had a date for the lumpectomy. And while my seventeen-year-old daughter burst into tears and immediately asked, "How do you know you won't get it again and die?" which I was not expecting, I was able to convince her, more or less, that I'd had a long conversation with a very good doctor who was sure I'd be just fine. Swathed in my own denial, I firmly believed there was no chance I would not be fine, and I think that made me more credible.

With Friends Like These . . .

Negativity has sharp, prickly edges that can pierce even a thick denial shield, so I did my utmost to avoid any situations where I might brush up against it. But every now and then you get caught unawares, blindsided by someone who means well but is, in the truest sense of the word, thoughtless.

I'm thinking of a man I met who had lost his beloved wife to breast cancer about a year earlier, and who, upon hearing that I had just been diagnosed, told me all about her long, sad struggle. I sat with him, trapped, listening to his story because I felt so bad for him, and he needed to talk, but I needed to escape, and I didn't. Luckily, because I am a world-class denier, he didn't scare me too much. As he was recounting his story, I was telling myself, "She was not stage one, she did not have a nice, early catch. She was not in your situation."

I wish I'd had the presence of mind to be more like Vivian McDevitt, a forty-seven-year-old breast cancer patient from New Jersey who had a double mastectomy. She refused to be around negativity of any kind, she told me at a book club meeting one evening. "You'll have a friend who had it and she had a bad time and she'll want to tell you all about her experience. I have literally said to people, 'Stop! I'm not interested in that information.'"

A young yoga instructor whom I've taken class with, Kelly Considine, was battling a recurrence of cancer when she was given a very hard time by some of her colleagues.

"They said if I were a vegan I wouldn't have cancer. I also got some flak about the chemo drugs I took. But who the hell are they to tell me what to do?"

Who, indeed. She was furious and hurt by the unsolicited advice, which also included the oh so helpful observation by a yoga teacher that if she had radiation, it would cause more cancer.

Even if you're lucky enough to duck the Debbie Downers of the world, it's pretty likely you'll be confronted with advice, whether you want it or not, whether you think the person dispensing it is full of crap or not.

Your friends and loved ones are going to have plenty to say. You'll find that some of them will be incredibly helpful, and others won't be, even though they think they are. It would be great if all of our friendships came with their own kind of Hippocratic oath: "First Do No Harm—and Second, Don't Say Something That Will Freak Her Out." Unfortunately, there's almost always some mostly well-meaning person who thinks, after watching enough episodes of *Oprah* and reading the right books, she is qualified to give you advice. The odds are pretty good that she's not, unless she's been through it either personally or alongside someone else at very close range, or is, in fact, an oncologist. You don't have to stand there and politely listen if you don't want to.

But if you are bombarded by friends and colleagues who want to tell you about the women they know who've also had breast cancer, here's a suggestion, one that I wish I'd thought of sooner. Ask them to call their friends to see whether they'd mind talking to you about their experiences. No one who's just found out she has breast cancer should be expected to cold-call a stranger to discuss such a personal topic, and if your friend really wants to help you she'll do this. (If not, do you need this gasbag in your life right at the moment? Maybe not.)

And for those of you who are friends of newly diagnosed breast cancer patients: Please, think twice before offering any advice that was not requested. Your friend/loved one is already being deluged with too much information. Don't volunteer your opinion, even if it's based on rock-solid knowledge, unless you're asked, and then, think hard about the effect it will have before answering.

Sometimes, "I don't know, do you want me to do some research for you on that?" is a better answer than the one you were about to give.

Mary Bryson, a professor at the University of British Columbia, who had breast cancer in 2007, had a blog called Big Grrls Do Cry. Here's some of what she said about the need to protect herself from some well-meaning friends in the early days after diagnosis and surgery:

"Any attempt to tell me (a) what it means to have cancer, as in, 'Cancer is a gift,' or (b) why I have cancer, as in, 'I know why you have cancer. It's the toxicity in your family,' are immediate grounds for exclusion. . . . People tend to be freaked out by the fact that there is precious little they can do to help me out. . . . And they can either coexist with that vulnerability, just like I have to, or they can't, in which case they will quickly slip away from the tangible landscape of my quotidian existence. I am good with it all."

You may have to let some well-meaning but toxic friends slip away from your landscape, at least while you're doing treatment. (And then, if you're really lucky, they won't come back when it's over.)

Breast Cancer Is Not the New Woodstock

Maybe because such a large proportion of breast cancer patients are baby boomers, some of my friends viewed my situation as just another generational experience, like the summer we all discovered tie-dye or something. Slightly more than a phase, but nothing to get too hung up about. I think this was part of our group denial, frankly. We all want to believe we'll live forever, and be forever young. Everybody regaled me with their tales of friends who breezed through breast cancer and now are back, "good as new." It was supposed to be calming to know that there are so damned many of us going through this nasty milestone, and that most of us are fine afterward. Too bad Fisher-Price doesn't make a My First Death Scare kit for grown-ups, with a doctor's bag, pink ribbons, and some toy breast implants. They'd just fly off the shelves.

Actually, it's because there are so many of us going through breast cancer that I knew the process of getting from here to there is a bitch. There was certainly little comfort in numbers. Think about it: When we were little kids lined up for shots, seeing the kids ahead of you getting stuck didn't make you any less likely to cry when it was your turn, did it? Or to be more than a little pissed off to find yourself trapped in this situation?

I remember feeling angry as I contemplated getting into that long line to treat my breast cancer (like all those other "kids"), but I didn't really know why I was angry then. Now, with some distance, I think I get it. I was just freakin' *enraged* that I was, officially, damaged goods, and there wasn't a bloody thing I could do to change that. In *Breast Cancer: Society Shapes an Epidemic*, the brilliant breast surgeon Dr. Susan Love describes it like this: "Once you are diagnosed with breast cancer you become an outsider. You no longer belong to the world of the 'temporarily immortal' but have joined the world of the 'defectives.'"

I didn't know it when I was going through it, but that truly is the crux of the issue. I just wanted to be the "real" me, an insider, not "an outsider." I was nowhere near ready to consider mortality, or even getting old. I didn't want to be pulled out of my posse, separated from my herd, cast off as a weakling. I wanted to run back to my life, my people, as if nothing had happened.

Wait for me, you guys, I'll be right back. Just gotta do this thing over here with the needles and the radiation for a minute . . . I'll catch up with you.

I did my best to avoid cold, harsh reality. It should be said, however, that as of now, 2 million women in America are going about our post–breast cancer lives. For the most part, even if we sometimes feel like factory seconds or re-conditioned merchandise, we're able to make a seamless transition back to our routines. Of course we are more aware of our mortality. The knowledge that cancer could return is like a low-level white noise in my head that suddenly gets loud every six months when I go for mammograms and sonograms. But once I get the "all clear" signal, I go straight back to living my life as I always did. I spend far too much time working, worrying about fat and wrinkles, and wishing I were having more fun.

Almost as if the whole thing never happened. Almost. Three years after treatment, my breast cancer seems both less real—like a bad dream whose details I'm eager to forget—and more real, in the sense that I've finally come to grips with the truths about it that I was incapable of handling while I was in the middle of treatment. All I can tell you is, I think I did the right thing for me. Fear is not helpful.

Take a deep breath, take your time, take human bites. And don't let anybody try to convince you that you can't "do" breast cancer your own way.

But you aren't going to do it all yourself, and you aren't going to do it alone.

A Lesson Not Learned from Breast Cancer

"True friends listen, offer support, and only give their opinions when asked . . . I get to make the decisions. If I want to eat peach pits and douse myself with holy water from Lourdes, it's my decision."

—Jeanne Sather, journalist, author of the blog

The Assertive Cancer Patient

Chapter Two

Delegate.
Don't Abdicate.

> **Lesson Two:**
>
> Even the biggest control freak
> has to let go and delegate
> responsibilities sometimes, and
> learning that you have cancer is
> one of those times. You are
> going to have to assemble a
> medical team with the express
> purpose of handing over
> control to them. But remember,
> they work for you.

I grew up as a middle child in a middle-class family in middle America. I got a middling education in the public schools, just like all the other baby boomer kids I knew. And mostly, what we learned of the world we learned from television.

We watched a lot of medical dramas—*Ben Casey, Dr. Kildare, Marcus Welby, M.D.* Ah, yes, it was the golden age of medicine. Doctors were omnipotent, patients were compliant, and nobody ever asked to see your insurance card before treating you.

Is it any surprise that we were all programmed to believe that Doctor Knew Best? (Our elderly parents, who were about the same age then that baby boomers are now, watched the same shows; far too often they *still* do what their doctors tell them, like docile lambs.)

And so when confronted with a serious diagnosis, maybe for the first time in our lives, we are torn between what we were taught then by popular culture and common practice, and what we know now about doctors.

We want the best doctor possible, and we know they aren't all equal, but who are we to determine?

Actually, it's not going to be that complicated. You just need to know what your personal priorities are.

It helps to focus just on the first task you face, which is to choose a surgeon. There will be other doctors, maybe a plastic surgeon, quite possibly an oncologist for chemo and a radiotherapist for radiation, but your surgeon will have some suggestions to help you with that part. You're going to have at least one or two meetings with these doctors. As intimidating as all of this is, it could be worse—much, much worse. We may be long past the days when a doctor would accept a plate of freshly baked brownies as payment for treating you, but be glad we aren't living in ancient Egypt, or mid-twentieth-century America.

The Good Doctor/The Good Patient:
In the Beginning

Women have known about and feared breast cancer for thousands of years. In fact, according to the Web site MedicineWorld.org, the first known description of breast tumors was written on Egyptian medical papyri sometime between 3000 and 1600 BC. (They recommended cauterizing for some kinds of tumors, using a tool called "the fire drill," but noted that there was no treatment.)

Hippocrates wrote of hard tumors in the breast in the fifth century BC. He was also credited with giving cancer its name: *karkinos*, which meant "crab" in Greek, because he thought tumors looked like crabs. He was right about a lot of his cancer observations, but totally wrong about what caused tumors, proving the wisdom of getting a second opinion, no matter how big a hotshot your doctor is.

Doctors began to perform mastectomies in the eighteenth century, which was long before anesthesia had been invented. The women were usually restrained—tied to chairs or bedposts. Among the poor women who suffered this hideous procedure was the French writer (and prefeminist feminist) Fanny Burney, whose mastectomy without anesthesia or antiseptic was performed by Napoleon's surgeon in 1811. That same year, the daughter of Abigail and John Adams endured a mastectomy at her parents' home in

Quincy, Massachusetts. At first, doctors thought the operation was a success. But it had come too late; the cancer had already spread and two years later Nabby Adams died.

For centuries, breast cancer patients tried all sorts of radical but ineffective treatments. As recounted in *Bathsheba's Breast* by James S. Olson, as recently as the 1950s there were doctors who, knowing that estrogen feeds tumors, would first do a radical mastectomy, then remove ovaries, then adrenal glands, and finally, in some advanced cases, the pituitary gland. It was a risky procedure that involved boring a hole into the patient's skull; Olson notes that some women suffered permanent vision impairment, personality changes, and a loss of cognitive functions. And these women were not uneducated, unsuspecting guinea pigs. They were upper-middle-class women with advanced breast cancers who put their faith in the all-powerful medical profession.

Obviously, things have changed, but maybe not enough. The journalist and blogger Jeanne Sather, who has been dealing with metastatic breast cancer for years, has a warning for women who have the urge to be the good patient:

"As you move along in your cancer treatment, you may be shocked to realize that you have been socialized, probably without realizing it, to be a 'good patient.' Good patients are cheerful, rarely complain (and may not give their doctors an accurate reading of their symptoms and problems as a result), and are hesitant to 'bother' the doctor—even when something is bothering *them.*

"As a result of not speaking up, these people not only don't get the best medical care, but they also may find their frustrations growing because their real concerns are not being expressed."

You Have the Right to Remain Loud

The women's health movement changed everything, and we all owe a great deal to the feminists who demanded the right to make informed choices about their own health care. In the thirty years since *Our Bodies, Ourselves* burst into the newly raised consciousness of America's women, the prospect of empowering patients to be involved in their medical treatments is no longer considered radical; it's the norm. It is, I believe, one of the only complete successes of the women's movement—we didn't get an equal rights amendment, we still don't earn equal pay for equal work, and reproductive rights are an ongoing battle. But women have fought for and won the right to have the final say about their medical treatment (and in doing so, won the same rights for men).

It's up to your doctor(s) to talk you through your options, and direct you to good resources where you can do your own research if you want to. This is not only what you have a right to expect, it may very well make you feel better.

Maybe you're thinking, *Yeah, well, I don't want to be in charge at this stage. What I really want is someone I can trust absolutely to take my hand, maybe even literally, and lead me.*

Fine. You can have that kind of doctor if you want, and lots of women do.

Choosing a doctor you can be comfortable with and totally trust is one of the most important decisions you have to make. And yet some of us are better prepared to meet with a cell phone salesman than we are to go into these doctors' appointments. Believe me, choosing a cell phone plan is far more confusing.

Who Do You Trust?

I've learned over the years that when confronting a new challenge, whatever it is, the first thing to figure out is what you don't know, and the second is to find the people who do know and are willing to help you. We women do that all the time, consulting one another on burning issues that range from "Can you recommend someone to test my son for a learning disability?" to "Do these jeans make me look fat?"

If you have a friend who's been through breast cancer, either personally or secondhand, don't be shy about calling her. You'll be surprised how many women will want to help you. I get calls and e-mails all the time from friends of friends, not because I'm any sort of expert—I'm not—but because I've been through it and have talked to so many other women who have been, too, and I'm glad to help if I can. We talk about doctors, facilities, great books to read, all kinds of helpful information.

Definitely call the doctor you trust the most, whether that's a gynecologist, an internist, or a family practitioner. They'll know who's got a great reputation in your community, and why. I always want to know who my doctor would choose for any procedure I'm about to have.

When I learned I had breast cancer, I didn't have any close friends who'd been through it (my, how that's changed!), but I was lucky to have a trusted resource, my gynecologist, Dr. Anne Carlon.

As I've said, she had called me almost immediately after I got the lab results. I wrote down what she was saying ("nice, early catch"), but I realized she was telling me more than I could process at that moment. Also, it was hard to hear her over the sound of my pounding heart and exploding head. I asked her if I could call her back later with questions, after I had finished freaking out and could think straight again, and of course she agreed.

When I called her back, an hour or so later, I wanted a list of doctors she could recommend. She gave me about ten names, several of whom were leading breast surgeons I'd heard of.

"If you had to choose for yourself, who would you pick?" I asked her. She mentioned a couple of names from the bigger list, including Dr. Rache Simmons, the doctor I ultimately chose.

Dr. Carlon has been with me through thick and thin and I trusted her implicitly. Still, rather than just go with her personal recommendation, I called the offices of each doctor on the list she'd given me, eliminating any doctor who couldn't see me for more than a week. Like many women, I made the mistake of believing that the most important thing was to act immediately. (How else could I meet my goal of having cancer "for twenty minutes")? Dr. Simmons is a great doctor with a superb reputation at an excellent medical practice, but in my panicky state, the fact that I could get an appointment with her within a week was almost as important as the fact that Dr. Carlon had recommended her.

And if you think I was a little crazed, recently I heard from a doctor who was visited by a woman with a very-early-stage breast cancer. The patient brought her husband, but she was a bundle of nerves. After the initial consultation, the husband asked if he might ask a few questions, and the doctor said, "Of course." But the patient turned to her husband and exclaimed, "While you're asking questions my cells are multiplying!"

I know just how she felt (it sounds like something I would have snapped at my slow-talking, deliberative husband), but if you ask your doctors, they'll tell you that you

46

have some time. Make the right decision, not the hastiest. I was very lucky to get the best of both worlds, a great doctor who could see me right away.

I also did a Google search on Dr. Simmons and read up on her before making the appointment. She was impressive, and it didn't hurt that she'd been profiled in the *Wall Street Journal* as a cutting-edge surgeon, no pun intended. Or that she'd been booked on *Good Morning America* and elsewhere to be the guest expert on breast cancer a few times.

When my husband, Dennis, and I arrived for my appointment and took two seats in the large yet strangely claustrophobic waiting room, I felt for the first time like I was in Cancertown. My stomach was in a tight ball and I made a mental note of the location of the ladies' room, just in case. The Breast Center occupies a whole floor of an office building, accommodating surgeons, oncologists, and a chemotherapy suite, and everywhere I turned, there were doors leading to somewhere I didn't want to be. As I looked around at the other patients waiting to see their doctors, I thought, *Nobody in this room is here for good news. Every one of these women has breast cancer.*

And yet still I managed to cling to the belief that I, alone among the women there, would have it relatively easy. (This was in the last moments before Dr. Simmons disabused me of the notion that I would not be having chemotherapy.)

We waited only a few minutes before being ushered into

her office—this was a big plus. I am almost pathologically impatient at doctors' offices. I hate it when they leave patients stacked up in examining rooms like planes over LaGuardia. I get resentful if the staff and doctor assume that I have nothing more important to do with my time than wait to be seen.

Oh, wait. I didn't.

Still, it's the principle of the thing.

I'll admit I did find Dr. Simmons a tad intimidating when we first met. She immediately struck me as wildly more competent than I could ever be. I mean, she was clearly supersmart, very attractive (she looks a little like Susan Sarandon), had really nice jewelry, and projected an aura of omnipotence without seeming arrogant. She radiated self-confidence; although, in all fairness, I would too if I looked like Susan Sarandon.

I was in the market for a terrific surgeon, and Dr. Simmons fit the bill. It was almost as if I had cast her to play the part of my breast surgeon. I was relieved to have found the right surgeon for me on the first try.

Before meeting Dr. Simmons for the first time, I assumed I would go for a second opinion elsewhere. I knew it was what I was *expected* to do. But later that day, when I was back home staring dully at the list of surgeons I'd compiled on the day of my diagnosis, it occurred to me that the second doctor might recommend things I didn't want to hear. What if he or she told me I should get a mastectomy, not a lumpectomy, as Dr. Simmons recommended? How was that going to be helpful to me?

It was one of the first ways I veered off the well-worn path of the breast cancer journey. I just didn't want to confuse myself with too many conflicting opinions, and since I liked the first one I'd received, getting a second opinion began to feel like a pointless gesture that you do just because everyone else is doing it, like buying a panini maker you'll never use.

So I opted to skip seeing another surgeon. Anyway, I trusted Dr. Simmons immediately, and based on the bit of research I'd done, what she told me about how she would approach my case matched up exactly with what I'd read. I also liked the fact that it was a full-service kind of practice, very well coordinated from the mammography to surgery, from the chemo treatment to radiation. They all talked to one another regularly, and that was very important to me. I went with my instincts and never regretted the decision to skip a second opinion.

Specifically, here are the characteristics I was looking for, and found, in Dr. Simmons:

1. She was direct and to the point without making me feel rushed.
2. She was up to speed on my case before I came in. She had my file in front of her and it was clear she'd read it and was prepared.

3. She was respectful of my questions, and didn't dismiss the research I'd done on my own as unworthy.

4. She treated me like a whole person——not just a tumor in a skirt. She talked to me while examining me, explaining what she was doing, and then also afterward, when I was fully dressed, in her office.

5. She had an excellent support staff who were friendly and helpful and incredibly nice.

6. She was brimming with experience and self-assurance, which made me feel confident and optimistic.

7. She had great credentials and came highly recommended.

They're traits that I think every great doctor will have. I'd look for most of those same traits in a great television producer, too, and believe me, I've known some producers who would be more than happy to do a thorough breast exam.

If you *do* get a second opinion, and it's quite different from the first, do you go to a third doctor for the tie-breaker? Yep, you might see a third, or who knows, even more, but in the end, you're going to have to choose the one you feel is most likely to respond to what you need. Experts in the field, though, say that all things being equal, tie goes to the doctor or team of doctors with the most experience handling your kind of cancer. That makes a lot of sense.

Searching for Dr. Right

So how do you prepare for a doctor's consultation?

This is an interview. You are asking the questions, and evaluating the doctor/candidate. I know, I know, it's hard to imagine how you can evaluate a doctor when he or she knows everything and you know virtually nothing about the subject. It's intimidating at a time when you are at your most vulnerable, which is one reason a lot of women ask more questions of their wedding planner than they do of a surgeon. It's also why it's an excellent idea to take another person in with you—your spouse, a friend, someone who can listen and take good notes.

If you've ever done an interview, though, you know that you need to have prepared questions in front of you. You need an agenda for the meeting.

I would suggest that before your first doctor's visit, you try to block out everything else on your mind, as best you can, and focus on planning this meeting. It will help you organize your brain and quiet your nerves if you create a list of the attributes you need in a doctor. For example, some women really feel strongly that they want only a woman surgeon, while others prefer a man. Do you want someone who'll basically just tell you what to do, or someone who lays out all your options and waits for you to decide? Whatever your unique preferences are, there is one attribute that you always want if you can get it, and again, that is experience. You want to be treated by doctors who have dealt with your particular situation many times. If you live in a small community that's some distance from a major cancer treatment center, consider whether you would be better off traveling to the big facility. It's shocking how often cancer patients fail to get all the treatment they should because of the inexperience or inadequacy of their health care providers. If you don't know where to go for advice about that, you can call the American Cancer Society (1-800-ACS-2345) or the National Cancer Institute, which has a list of hospitals it designates as having excellent records, at 1-800-4-CANCER. Or go to their Web site at www.cancer.gov.

When I was calling the names Dr. Carlon had given me, some were men and some were women. I preferred a woman, but I think it would have been fine if I'd gone with a dude. I did want a doctor who would explain my options to me and then let me make up my own mind about treatment.

The huge mistake I made was in misunderstanding the amount of insurance coverage I actually had, and what it meant in real terms to have a cap on out-of-pocket expenses. My insurance was through Air America, and it sucked (although we were probably lucky to have even crappy insurance, given our financial state at that time). I had many, many uncovered expenses, and I am fortunate to have generous parents who helped me pay some large bills.

When you've made your list of dream date doctor characteristics and you move on to the questions you want to ask, please—make sure you understand your insurance coverage, and don't be embarrassed to ask the doctor what coverage she or he accepts. You also need to get the insurance company on the phone to let them know what's going on before you begin any kind of treatment. Get the name of the person you're dealing with. This is a good time to have someone else with you to listen in on your conversation and pay attention to the answers. You may find yourself in a battle or two or three with your insurance company about what they're agreeing to pay for. You will not be in your best shape to fight them (do you think they know that? I do), so having an advocate who's tenacious and relentless will help you a lot.

As for the medical questions you'll want to ask, the odds are you don't even know what you don't even know, but you can consult any number of Web sites to find out. I like breastcancer.org and www.cancer.gov.

Obviously, you want to know what the doctor can tell you about your cancer: what is the stage, what are your treatment options, will the doctors test a sentinel node to see whether cancer cells have reached your lymph nodes, what kind of testing will be done on the tumor—for example, will they do the oncotype DX test that helps determine whether or not you would benefit from chemo-therapy? These are just a few of the questions you'll want to ask. Many others will have to wait until after you've had surgery.

I'd say that if your prospective surgeon doesn't want to be asked a lot of questions, that tells you a lot, right there.

When the Doctor Is Not McDreamy

I went to an internist once who clearly wanted to be on television and wasn't so much examining me as he was auditioning for me. In a social situation it wouldn't have bothered me so much, but I was lying on an examining table at the time, covered only by a thin cloth, and he was pawing at all my vital organs. After that, how the hell would I ever be able to share a cup of joe with him in the green room before a TV appearance? I never went back, nor did I ever book him as a guest expert.

Sometimes you just know right away that you and a doctor are wrong for each other. The television news-woman Linda Ellerbee certainly knew that when she was diagnosed with breast cancer. She said in an interview in *Prevention* magazine: "The surgeon I went to initially said, 'You have so many questions. Why don't you read a book by a doctor named Susan Love? Then you won't have to annoy me.' That's a direct quote. I told him I would not only get her book—I'd ask her to do my surgery. And she did."

Linda has been a hero of mine for years. She clearly did not allow herself to get sucked into the "good girl syndrome" that many women, even seemingly powerful ones, get all hung up on. I don't know why so many of us have the desperate-to-please trait. Could it be a remnant from trying to please the first towering authority figures in our lives, our dads? Those of us who were determined to impress Daddy in some cases certainly transferred that impulse to our mostly-male bosses and pretty much all authority figures, and when you have cancer, let's face it, your doctor is the ultimate authority figure. You are small and helpless and she or he is big and all-powerful. I had a bad case of Daddy/boss syndrome off and on for years. It wasn't cured until I had a spectacularly awful boss—a big man-baby who I concluded fairly quickly would be impossible to please, and not worthy of the effort. It was incredibly liberating to realize that I did not have to measure myself against his expectations, which changed constantly, anyway. That realization has helped me with all authority figures, including doctors.

My friend Fiona Conway, a television news executive, almost got caught in the good-girl web herself. She had been diagnosed with stage II breast cancer, and we had lunch shortly after she'd interviewed several oncologists. I was shocked to hear her describe her experience with the first doctor, a man who conveyed nothing but negativity to her.

"He held my file and said, 'This is tough. Very worrisome,'" she said. "He was shaking his head. He also said it was a stage three, until I insisted that he check out my pathology reports again. And even then, he was reluctant to say that it was actually stage two cancer."

She was, of course, deeply upset by the encounter. But as she replayed it in her mind, over and over during a long holiday weekend, she kept trying to justify his behavior. She rationalized that he was probably just trying to be honest with her and tried to convince herself she could get used to his manner. Fiona is incredibly smart and assertive and knows how to get what she needs, wherever in the world she finds herself. Her instinct told her this guy was absolutely wrong for her, but she *still* tried to convince herself it was her problem, not his. If it wasn't a case of good girl syndrome, it had to be breast cancer–induced timidity, a very common condition, but one that is curable, fortunately. The cure is to listen to what your gut is telling you, which is what I told her when she asked for my advice. (I wanted to scream, "Are you fucking kidding me? Don't you dare go back to him," but I didn't. What if she had chosen him, and knew I thought it was an awful idea? It would be just like a friend who breaks up with a guy, and you tell her how all her friends hated him, and then six months later she's gotten back with him and they're getting married. You can kiss that friendship good-bye.) Still, I did strongly suggest that she could find a doctor who was more simpatico with her. As she later acknowledged, that was what she wanted to hear.

The next week she met with another doctor who told her he believed she'd be fine, which of course was an immense relief to her. Ultimately, because the second doctor was in New York and she lives in New Jersey, she went with a third doctor, Dr. Bonni Gearhart, who has been reassuring, incredibly skillful, and a lot of fun to talk to.

I've found Dr. Gearhart, whom I have consulted about a number of questions for this book, to be a force of positive energy. She believes it's up to her, as the oncologist, to understand the kind of woman her patient is, and to adapt her bedside (and office-side) manner accordingly. Not every doctor is that adept, but you at least want them to *get* you, and what you need. It's not up to you to become the kind of patient you think your doctor wants you to be.

You have enough to worry about; you don't need to be worrying about whether you're living up to a doctor's expectations. Kyle Good, who is a vice president at Scholastic, Inc., had the horrible situation of discovering she had breast cancer while her husband was in a late stage of melanoma. She had surgery, but when she consulted one of the top breast cancer doctors in the world, she would not accept his advice to go through chemotherapy. Telling this doctor you disagree with him is like telling Wolfgang Puck he ought to use more salt. The doctor was very firm, but so was Kyle. She had a young son, and couldn't imagine how he would deal with having two parents on chemo. Kyle saw another top oncologist with impressive credentials, who agreed that she could forgo chemo if they kept a close watch on her. It's been ten years now, and Kyle's fine.

Different Folks for Different Strokes

Because you will have to choose several doctors, it's important to remember that you need different things in different situations. For example, when I'm nervous, like, say, when someone is telling me I have cancer, I tend to make a lot of jokes. Often, nobody laughs, but it doesn't stop me from inappropriately cracking wise. It's sort of my own variety of Tourette's syndrome, and, considering my vocabulary for off-color words, I guess it could be worse.

Anyway, in post-surgery visits, I cracked a lot of stupid jokes when I was in Dr. Simmons's office. I'm not sure she ever laughed at a single one of them; she would smile politely, just to be nice, and that would remind me to let her do her job and stop trying to entertain her with tortured jokes that weren't funny to anybody. I didn't need my surgeon to find me amusing; I needed her to get me tumor-free, and she did.

On the other hand, the doctor who would see me through months of chemo had to be somebody who did truly understand my warped sense of humor at a time when I was a nervous, sometimes cranky control freak.

Dr. Ellen Chuang, my oncologist, was a good audience as

well as a great doctor, which I really needed during the long months of the crapathon that is chemo. She was very collaborative about the various decisions we had to make. She never made me feel vain or silly about any of the arguably superficial issues that concerned me. I knew we'd get along just fine.

Sometimes You Don't Get a Vote . . .

After slowly learning all about the details of the first part of my treatment, the lumpectomy, I was nervous but clear-headed when I went to the preoperation meeting with Dr. Simmons the day before my surgery. I had enough information to know that as procedures go, it wouldn't be that tough. I'd been through a partial hysterectomy, root canal, and childbirth. I could do this.

I also met that day with the radiation oncologist to learn about an innovative procedure called mammosite therapy, in which a kind of balloon is surgically inserted into the empty space created by the removal of the tumor and surrounding breast tissue. Radiation "seeds" are delivered into the balloon through a catheter, and then removed after the treatment session. The mammosite stays in for a week, and the patient goes in twice a day for treatments, but then, you're done. So instead of six or seven long weeks of daily radiation, you get it over with in five days. I thought that was a great idea and enthusiastically agreed. "See," I told my husband as we drove home. "I knew this wasn't going to be that bad."

Of course, even the best laid plans sometimes come out differently than you expect. But that's what happens when, as team leader, you delegate some responsibility to others.

As the executive producer of two different network morning shows, there were many nights I went to bed with a clear idea of what the next day's program was going to be, only to learn in the wee hours of the morning that breaking news, or other circumstances, required producers to change my plans overnight. That was their job; I had delegated that responsibility to them. And I trusted them to use good judgment.

It only took me about twenty-five years to learn how to let go, but eventually I did come to understand that you just can't be in control of every detail, every minute, whether you're talking about a live report out of Baghdad or, in the case of my breast cancer surgery, a little hiccup in my lumpectomy procedure.

Before surgery, I had decided that when I woke up I was going to deliver the line Ronald Reagan made famous in the film *King's Row*: "Where's the rest of me?" he shouts as he wakes up in a hospital room to find his legs have been amputated.

I thought it would be so clever and witty. So very me to wake up and tell a joke.

Instead, when I woke up, I soon found myself crying, not laughing. As I came out of the anesthesia, I ran my fingers along my right side for the tube connected to the mammosite implant. It wasn't there. The nurse told me my doctors had not implanted that great new radiation delivery system after all. Something about it not fitting. Immediately, hot tears spurted into my eyes. The nurses hastily assured me that conventional radiation is not so bad (which is true), but that wasn't the point. I had made a decision about treatment and I had gone under the anesthesia knowing what to expect when I came to. Instead, while I was out, I was overruled.

God, how I hate it when that happens, whatever the reason. You see, I *know* I have to delegate, but on an emotional level it stings, even when the reason I've been overruled is perfectly valid and for my own good.

I was feeling that sting when I woke up from surgery. Yes, I had given my medical team the responsibility to use their best judgment, and I trusted that they had made the right call. It wasn't rational, and I knew it. In retrospect, I think that one invalidated decision became the focus of my anger about having to go through all of this in the first place. And, as Dr. Gearhart has reminded me, doctors don't know yet if mammosite will prove over time to be as effective as standard radiation. It may be that my big disappointment was a blessing in disguise.

For more than a week, every time I looked at my swollen, bruised, and stitched-up breast I was reminded how powerless I had been. I felt assaulted. I walked around for days resisting the urge to pull up my shirt and shout, "Look what they did to me!" to anybody who'd listen.

(By the way, Jessica Stedman Guff had the mammosite implant, and while she was glad she did, she said it was very uncomfortable. "I have new respect for Pamela Anderson," she joked.)

There is nothing wrong with being angry or sad or bitter, if that's how you're feeling. I think it would be far worse to tell yourself you shouldn't get down, when you already are. It's awful to have your emotions negated.

When you're feeling the need to shake off a bad mood, at any stage of your treatment, you may find it helpful and calming to stop and ask yourself what is most important to your recovery at that moment. What do you need, right now, to feel better, both physically and emotionally? And then ask for it, explicitly. Don't feel that you're being a burden or a baby or a bitch. Your doctors, remember, are supposed to be working for you, not the other way around. But they're not mind readers. And neither, by the way, are your friends or family.

. . . But It Feels Great When You Do Get a Vote

After surgery, when I was meeting with Dr. Chuang to talk about further treatment, I had all kinds of questions that had nothing to do with curing cancer, per se. For example, I wanted to know if I would still be able to get Botox. Also, whether I could dye my hair if I had a chemotherapy that didn't make it all fall out. (I saw no point in keeping my hair if it was going to be gray.) I wanted to know if I could still go to work. And I wanted to know if I would gain weight or lose weight, and if that was controllable. She seemed a bit surprised by a few of my questions, but she listened, and gave me what I considered to be the right answers, which included a green light to color my hair if I had hair. We set the date to begin chemo. Now all I had to do was decide which kind of chemo to choose, and I had some weeks to think about it.

You delegate responsibility, but you don't abdicate your role as the team leader. And what I know, after being a team leader for many years, in many different situations, is that what people want most is a clear understanding of your wishes, and a strategy to execute your plan.

But there has to be room for adjustment, if necessary. And I was feeling a little too penned in. We had agreed on a plan for starting my chemotherapy, but it just wasn't sitting right with me. You'd think I'd have realized, as a person whose main place of business for years was a Control Room, that what I needed to feel like myself again was to take back some control over my life. Unfortunately, I didn't realize that, and walked around for weeks feeling intermittently angry and a bit depressed. Part of the problem was also that I'd had to cancel a trip to Italy, which was very disappointing.

The more I thought about it, the madder I got. What I needed was to get my bossy-girl mojo back. I wanted control. And I wanted to go to Italy.

I asked Dr. Chuang if we could delay the scheduled start of chemotherapy for a few weeks so that my family could take the trip we'd planned before my summer got screwed up by breast cancer. She counted out the weeks, gave me a date by which I absolutely had to begin treatment, and off we went to Umbria and Tuscany.

Delegate, Schmelegate: It's Your Kids' World. You're Just Barfing in It.

Although our trip had been planned long before I found out I had breast cancer, I couldn't have chosen a better place to go on vacation before chemotherapy. The Italians really know how to enjoy life. There's natural beauty, art, great food and wine, and a pace that forces you to slow down and enjoy it. It was perfect.

Sort of. The truth is that while we had a wonderful trip, there was a lot of pressure on everybody to have One Last Good Time for a while. At first that sentiment was unspoken, then it was quietly articulated, and finally, it was snarled, all by me, all at our teenaged daughter, Julia, who just didn't want to deal with my expectations. Looking back on it, she thinks I was a little too convincing when I told her not to worry and insisted that she not treat me differently. She definitely didn't ease up on the parent-teenager drama. (Usually, when we traveled with Julia she brought a friend, but this time it was just the three of us. Silly me, I thought it would be good to have some intimate family time.)

Instead, there was sulking at the Borghese Gardens in Rome, a meltdown in Perugia, a snarkfest in Todi. I will admit to being surprised by my daughter in Italy; she is normally a considerate and empathetic kid. She was with us at the hospital the day I had surgery and was helpful in the days afterward. But the pressure to Have a Meaningful Experience in Italy may have been too much. It all came to a head one day in the lovely town of Assisi, home of St. Francis. I had been lingering over silk headbands at some little shop, and when she asked me why, I told her I was thinking of getting a few for when my hair was thin from chemo.

"Stop talking about cancer," she barked loudly at me. "I don't want to hear about it anymore." (Was I talking about it a lot? I thought I barely mentioned it; she says I mentioned it constantly. In any case, it was clearly too much for her.)

I have since learned, from all the moms I've interviewed for this book, that kids have their own way of dealing with the fear that comes with your diagnosis. Sometimes they're unbelievably sweet and thoughtful, and sometimes they seem unfathomably selfish. Julia was mostly sweet and thoughtful, but she had her fearful moments. Teenagers in particular are tough; their emotions are so raw under the best of circumstances. Having a mother with breast cancer upsets their fragile equilibrium and forces them to confront one more thing to worry about, one more situation that sets them apart from their friends, one more problem that's out of their control.

Still, I believe kids want to make some kind of contribution, and since this chapter began with a discussion about delegating responsibility without giving up authority, I would suggest you ask your kids how they want to pitch in. Little ones may be more than eager to help you. Teenagers, while guarding their routines as much as possible, probably will also want to feel the sense of empowerment that is a by-product of responsibilities. Julia was a sympathetic and helpful daughter once I began the chemo and had days of feeling kind of lousy.

A former colleague of mine recently discovered she had breast cancer. She told me how her three kids, a college freshman, a sixteen-year-old son, and a fourteen-year-old daughter, were dealing with her situation. Her eldest was concerned, and her middle son was very worried about her, but her daughter, after being very upset when she first got the news, went through a period when she seemed curiously unmoved (of course, you have to consider that fourteen-year-old girls are more or less clinically insane anyway and can't be held responsible for all of their actions). She refused to talk about it. Fortunately, my friend retained her wicked sense of humor.

"Finally, the other night she came into my room and

sat down on my bed, sobbing," her mother told me. "I said, 'Oh, honey, it's okay. I'm so glad you're ready to talk about your feelings. Tell me what's going through your head.' "

"Mom, I really need a horse," her daughter wailed through the tears.

We howled over that, but not as much as when she told me that her middle son had promised to shave his head in solidarity with her when she loses her hair to chemo.

"We announced that the whole family was doing it. You should have seen her face when she thought she'd have to shave her long, thick hair, too." (Eventually, they told her daughter she was off the hook. In the end, she was very helpful and supportive to her mother.)

What looks like indifference may well be fear. I've come to think that talking to your kids about breast cancer is a lot like talking to them for the first time about sex. There's a limit to how much information they can handle at one time. If you pay attention, you'll know when they've taken in as much as they can in one sitting. Let them take human bites, too.

The very wise Ann Pleshette Murphy, who is *Good Morning America*'s parenting expert, suggests that you be as honest with your kids as possible. She also has a great technique for finding out how much they can handle.

"When they ask you a tough question, about cancer or anything else, sometimes it's best to ask them back, 'What do you think is the answer?' That way you find out what they're thinking and you can respond without overwhelming them."

And remember that when it comes to kids, it's their world, and we're just barfing in it.

A Lesson Not Learned from Breast Cancer

"What I already knew before having breast cancer was the importance of understanding your digestive system. I've paid attention to what my system needs since I was in my twenties. It's critical to your health. That means, when you have breast cancer, that you literally have to pay attention to everything you put in your mouth from the moment you're diagnosed. Because I knew what I needed, chemo wasn't that difficult for me."

—Vivian McDevitt

Chapter Three

Trust Your Inner Voice

*"If you live without awareness it is the same as dead.
You cannot call that kind of existence being alive."*

—Thich Nhat Hanh, Buddhist master,

from No Death, No Fear

Until you've been through cancer treatment, either for yourself or someone close to you, you probably think that from the minute they find a tumor until the minute your treatment is over, your medical team is in nonstop action. Cut it, poison it, zap it. In fact, that's not the case at all. It turns out there's a lot of waiting-around time, while you're waiting for pathology reports and your doctors are treating other patients, and it can be the hardest time to deal with emotionally. You don't see this depicted in documentaries or movies because there's no grand dramatic action for a camera to pick up.

Perhaps the one place where a whole lot is happening is in your head. We all have the inner voice that guides us—call it instinct, call it intuition, call it Terry the Talking Tumor (okay, maybe not that)—but whatever you call it, at the end of the day, when all the other voices are gone, that's the one you hear loud and clear. My inner voice is far from perfect, and sometimes I reject what it's telling me, but over the years it has earned my trust, and I will always at least consider what it's trying to say.

It's something I learned not from breast cancer but from my job. I had to make a zillion decisions every day. Some of them were no-brainers. But sometimes I agonized over whether to do a particular story or book a particular guest. It might be good for ratings, but was it good for the social discourse, or the image of whatever show I was producing at the time? (Believe it or not, I really did think about those things, which is probably why I'm no longer executive producing television shows.)

Sometimes it wasn't a question of if we'd tell a story, but how. I was producing *Good Morning America* during the Monica Lewinsky saga, and there were way too many mornings when I had to figure out whether, or how, to tell certain tawdry details of the story while taking into consideration that young kids might be watching with their parents. At *GMA* and then years later at CNN, there seemed to be an almost unlimited supply of tabloid stories, good for nothing but ratings, that I might feel pressured to pencil into a show while holding my nose.

Eventually I learned that if the little voice inside my head was telling me I was going to hate myself for doing something, it was best to listen, not for my career but for my peace of mind. The rule applies to all kinds of decisions I have to make in everyday life. If I go ahead and do something against my better judgment, it makes my stomach hurt. My inner voice must live in my stomach.

Whatever you call it, your inner voice can be your compass through breast cancer treatment, if you let it; in other words, if you trust yourself.

Do Something

While I was recovering from surgery before beginning the next phase of treatment, my inner voice wasn't exactly whispering.

In fact there were big, loud, endless debates going on in my head as I waited for the pathology reports to tell us all the details about my breast cancer. I knew the doctors would probably recommend chemotherapy, and I wanted to be prepared to make the right decision.

I could have simply waited patiently for the results

and then dealt with the various options, except that sitting around and waiting patiently is not what I do. I invariably ignore people who tell me "there's nothing to do now but wait," no matter what the circumstances. I believe it's always better to do something than to do nothing, so during the limbo between my lumpectomy and the lab results coming in, I was reading everything I could about chemotherapy.

I was online night and day, obsessing about what I might have to deal with: "If it's X, I'll need to do Y, but if it's Y, I should think about Z." Suddenly, it was as if I were reliving ninth-grade algebra, and that was at least as scary as breast cancer. I never could "solve for X."

It got awfully loud in my head.

Kelly Considine, a young, lithe yoga instructor, described the period between discovering cancer and beginning treatment as "like having a news ticker that's always running across my brain, displaying the words 'you've got cancer.' I go about my life and try to act normal but really, I can't think about anything else."

Six months after completing treatment for a stage II cancer she'd spent a year trying to get rid of, Kelly had a recurrence.

"When you're in the middle of treatment, you've got a team of doctors working with you and you put your head down and do what has to be done. It's actually scarier when it's all over, or in my case, when I'm waiting to begin all over again."

Beware the Attitude Police

Those waiting times are frustrating and anxiety-provoking. This is when fears and doubts creep in, even as people you know exhort you to keep a positive attitude, and fight the good fight.

Well, duh. Nobody thinks, *Screw it. I'm going to be depressed and negative until this thing is over.* We all *want* to be strong and brave and have a positive attitude, but what about those days when you just aren't feeling it? You can end up worrying that you're somehow failing as a "soldier" and will not only disappoint your loved ones but will also cause your cancer to grow.

Death by Bad Attitude. Smile or else, baby.

I suspect a lot of the positivity pushing is the product of well-meaning but unimaginative friends who don't know what else to say, yet feel obliged to say something.

(Hint to those people: Try listening instead of talking.)

You know when I have a negative attitude? When I hear someone say something like, "There's no such thing as incurable disease, only incurable people," and that generally "happy people don't get sick." That's the message of people like the famous, much-beloved bestselling author Dr. Bernie Siegel.

Gosh, it's a wonder I've lived as long as I have, cranky chick that I am sometimes.

I know that many people are comforted by Dr. Siegel and others like him who say that you can control your health with your mind. Me, not so much.

Maybe, if I were a Vulcan or something, that would be true. But if my brain could control my body, I would be five feet eight, a size two, and eat as much fatty food as I wanted. It should be a lot easier to mentally jack up my metabolism than to find and destroy cancer cells, but I haven't been able to do a thing for my metabolism, so I'm going to assume that I can't control cancer cells with the power of positive thinking, either.

Besides, if I do have the power to heal myself with a good mental attitude, doesn't that suggest that I also had the power to cause my illness through negative thoughts? Blaming the victim, in other words, for her own illness. I don't accept that.

I mean, think about it. Do you really believe any random cancer cells are taking note of your outlook on life before deciding whether to metastasize or die? I agree with the late, great, and much missed political columnist Molly Ivins, who died of inflammatory breast cancer in 2007.

As she wrote in a 2002 article in *Time*, "I suspect that cancer doesn't give a rat's ass whether you have a positive mental attitude. It just sits in there multiplying away, whether you are admirably stoic or weeping and wailing. The only reason to have a positive mental attitude is that it makes life better. It doesn't cure cancer."

Anyway, positive thinkers get cancer, too.

Gloria (who prefers I not use her last name) is one of the sunniest, most positive people I know. And yet, she was diagnosed with breast cancer in July of 2006, just months after her mother completed treatment for it. It was a shock to her, and a heartbreak to her mother, but she was upbeat when she told me the news. She was certain she'd get through her treatment and be fine.

Sounds like the right attitude, doesn't it? But, in fact, she had an awful time, emotionally and physically.

"Chemo kicked my ass," she told me when it was all over. "I was too weak and sick to work, so I was home all day, depressed, just watching TV. I would cry over a commercial. Anything could set me off."

Not exactly the optimal frame of mind for fighting cancer, huh? And yet, if you saw her today, you'd see a beaming, healthy, happy woman.

In fact, there is no scientific evidence that proves a connection between attitude and survival. For decades, researchers have done a variety of studies to see whether the people with cancer who have positive attitudes and a fighting spirit actually live longer than those who are fatalistic or felt helpless or hopeless. In a report published in the *British Medical Journal* in November 2002, which analyzed twenty-eight previous studies, doctors had to conclude that there is no direct relationship between your attitude and your survival.

To say that there is flies in the face of the facts and can freak out women who have enough to worry about without having to feel like a failure at Attitude Camp.

Here's what I think about all that "keep a positive attitude" talk:

If it's what you tell yourself, because it seems helpful and is something you feel you can do, that's great. But oncology psychiatrists will tell you that you have to let yourself have cranky "cancer days" when the spirit moves you, and not worry about it if you do. Everybody feels crappy sometimes, and if you get a little weepy or you feel sorry for yourself, it's no big deal. Don't stress about it.

A psychiatrist at Memorial Sloan-Kettering, Dr. Jimmie Holland, calls this "the tyranny of positive thinking."

On the other hand, while your attitude is not relevant to your long-term prognosis, it *is* extremely relevant to how you feel. A positive attitude will probably get you to do things that are good for your health. The oncologist Dr. Bonni Gearhart points out that if you're keeping a positive outlook, "you'll probably eat better, exercise more, get out and interact with other people more, and even notice when there are changes in your body you need to pay attention to. A better attitude can certainly lead to better health."

And when you're doing something to help yourself, whatever it is, you are surely more likely to feel empowered, which is good for the spirit. So do something. Do whatever it is you do to make yourself feel better. If you believe in God, pray. If you believe in science, do some research. If you're a gal who likes to hedge her bets, pray to God that the science works.

Here's a bit of advice I hope will be constructive: The minute someone tells you to cheer up when you just don't feel cheerful, or that you absolutely have to keep a positive attitude if you want to beat cancer, close your eyes and visualize yourself mooning him. It will make you smile and it will make him think you're actually doing as he suggests. It also lets you answer, "Oh, yes!" if you're ever asked by the attitude police whether you use the power of visualization to help yourself heal.

(And it proves that, by not telling him just to bug off and leave you alone, you clearly don't have that nasty, negative "cancer personality" in the first place.)

The journalist Jeanne Sather, of The Assertive Cancer Patient blog, has an interesting take on other people's expectations:

"I think that the people surrounding a person living with cancer often need that person to be a superhero. They don't want to see you frightened, or sad, or depressed. I try to deal with these expectations as best I can, even if it means that I no longer see some people, the most extreme way of dealing with them."

I was glad that none of my friends or family tried to offer advice about what I "should" do. I did have a friend who told me she was praying for me, which I found kind of upsetting. I didn't think my condition required divine intervention, and I believed she was praying to make herself feel better—so why tell me about it? I know there are millions of people who believe in the power of prayer, but I'm not one of them (which she knew, by the way). I wanted to be gracious about what was meant to be a gesture of kindness, but it felt more like a vote of no confidence in me. And, geez, if you can't be crabby when you've got the big C, when can you be? Eventually, she (and several others who made the same mistake of telling me they were praying for me) either stopped doing it or just stopped telling me they were.

The Miracle of Mindfulness Eludes Me

The fact that I'm not a religious person, that I don't look to God to solve my problems, doesn't mean that I wouldn't *like* to be a spiritual person. And I certainly know I'm in the minority in this regard. Almost everybody in this country believes in God, and, according to a Gallup poll in June 2007, 75 percent of Americans also believe in the existence of angels. This would be an astonishing statistic to me, were it not for the fact that wherever you go on breast cancer Web sites, somebody is trying to sell you an angel.

I have often contemplated what it would be like to have an angel watching over me. It seems like a nice idea at first, but then I get to wondering: Does the angel watch you all the time? Like, when you're doing private things you don't even like your dog to see you doing? It just feels wrong to me. I live in Manhattan; if I want someone constantly watching over me, I can just raise the shades and let some creepy guy across the way get a good eyeful.

The other thing about guardian angels is, if you do believe in them and they're supposed to be protecting you, where the hell were they when you were getting cancer?

I hate to say it, but if you had a guardian angel before you got breast cancer, apparently that angel was a fuckup. Or at the very least, out having a smoke or sleeping late or something, and therefore kind of a slacker.

During my search for usable information about chemotherapy, I kept finding angels for sale on breast cancer Web sites. And not just angels. Fairies, too.

I don't know where fairies land on the spiritual ladder, but judging from their increasing presence on Web sites I look at, it seems that those of us who battle serious diseases are practically being overrun with them. If Lou Dobbs weren't so concerned with Mexicans sneaking across our borders, he'd probably do a big exposé about fairies. I'm especially curious about a lovely Web site where all the fairies look like Santa Claus. The Web site, in fact, appears to be inspired by Christmas, not cancer, thankfully, but they do have a Spirit of Hope fairy for breast cancer (bendable and posable, three different sizes) that's all dressed up in . . . wait for it . . . pink. He just looks like Santa in pink instead of red (white beard, twinkly eyes, and so on), and some of the proceeds go to breast cancer research. I looked at this Santa-like dude in pointy shoes and thought, *Hey, Santa, it was supposed to*

*be a lump of coal in my stocking, not a lump in my . . . oh,
the hell with it.*

You learn the strangest things on the Internet when all
you're trying to do is find some facts about chemotherapy.
But without key bits of pending information from pathology
reports, and also a medical degree, I was only making myself crazy as I scoured the Web, trying to educate myself.

Eventually I abandoned the quest for knowledge about
cancer and switched to a quest for knowledge about my
spiritual self. This was during the peak of my misconcep-
tion about what the experience would be all about for me. I
was still assuming that at some point I was going to be enriched by some life-changing insight.

Ignoring the voice in my head that was saying, "You?
Spiritual? Really?" I decided to go on the search for insight
in an angels- and fairies-free zone.

I had once been taken to hear a lecture by the Viet-
namese Buddhist monk Thich Nhat Hanh, and although
I was surrounded by so many celebrities I felt like a seat
warmer at the Oscars, I found his powerful message of
peace and awareness to be truly inspirational. I left feeling
both uplifted and deeper at the same time. It seemed like a
spiritual awakening, but the truth is my spirit was asleep
again by the time I got home.

Still, I had high hopes that if I spent more time con-
templating the Buddhist philosophy of life through Nhat
Hanh, he might be my spiritual guide through breast cancer. I began reading one of his books, *No Death, No Fear.*

No help.

I highly recommend reading it now; on the topic of "life without limit" and in his poem to recite to the dying, the simple beauty of his writings can move me to tears.

But at that time, as I was in a kind of controlled panic over what the hell do I do now, I found that what I wanted was literal guidance, not spiritual. Nhat Hanh speaks frequently of mindfulness, and I was mindful of the fact that I just couldn't slow down, breathe, and delve that deeply with him, not at that moment.

It was as if there were a firewall stopping me from any kind of introspection about what I was going through. Yes, I questioned whether this meant I was a shallow, spiritually impoverished person. But what was really happening was self-protection. This was not the time to plumb the depths of my emotions or to discover what I really thought about the notion of no birth, no death, no self; I needed to square my shoulders, lower my head, and just push on. Move forward, as Christopher Reeve used to say.

I think my spiritual journey to learn the meaning of breast cancer lasted one weekend.

Zen and the Art of Internet Searching

My inner voice reminded me that, cosmically speaking, I was more at one with the World Wide Web than I was with the world, so I went back online. This time I found the True Path to Knowledge about breast cancer by searching more consumer-oriented, general info Web sites. And by that I mean Web sites that were written for people who are neither scientists nor spiritualists.

My enlightenment came from good sources like Mamm. com (the breast cancer magazine's Web site), breastcancer.org, Susanlove.com, and several others, where I learned that while I couldn't make decisions yet and shouldn't try, I could get educated about the terms I would need to understand when the lab results came back.

Instead of trying to learn everything about the various kinds of chemo decisions I might be faced with, this time I limited myself to trying to learn the terminology I would soon hear from my surgeon when she had all the facts about my tumor. I made a vocabulary list of key phrases and terms, and a subset of questions from that. Stages, tumor grades, HER-2/neu negative or positive, estrogen receptor negative or positive—none of those terms meant anything to me before, but now it was going to be vital that I understand them well enough to ask intelligent questions.

If you're going to do research on the Web, here's something you need to remember: It's crucial that you make sure the information you're reading is up-to-date. Lots of times you'll run across something that seems authoritative, and it probably was, back when it was originally published. But now, it may be way past its expiration date. It's also important to know who the source of the information is. Does the author have a financial stake or some other vested interest? And is the site written by well-credentialed people?

I didn't think for a second that my vocabulary list was complete, and it wasn't, but at least I was doing something to prepare myself. I was being me. (True, I was doing it at my office when I was supposed to be paying attention to other things, but, hey, sometimes that's me, too.)

A Different Kind of Revelation:
Fear of Chat Rooms

I made another mistake during this limbo period, one that I repeated several times during other stages before I got it through my thick head that this was not something that worked for me.

Chat rooms. I visited several of them, looking for on-line support. Weren't chat rooms a required part of the trip, a rest stop on the road of my breast cancer journey to a better me?

The truth is, chat rooms were a disaster for me. They filled my head with the stories of women who were scared and angry and felt just terrible. They needed a safe place to complain or ask questions or seek reassurance, and they had every right to, but they were not the voices I wanted to hear. They frightened me. They weakened my resolve and made me question whether I was nuts to think I would get through breast cancer and just resume my life.

This may sound like harsh talk to some in the pink bubble of the cancerocracy, but I promise you, there are plenty of women who fear and avoid the chat rooms for the same reasons I did. We all have to do whatever we can to get ourselves through this traumatic, awful time, without judging each other.

If you do go to a chat room, keep tabs on how it's affecting your mood. Maybe just drop in for a visit, without logging in or registering, to get a sense of the lay of the land. There is a lot of useful information on some sites, but if you're going to pay a high emotional price to find it, you may well be better off going to a site that is purely informational.

I look at it this way. If a friend or acquaintance calls me because she has breast cancer and wants to compare notes and get my opinion, I never, ever tell her things that I think would scare her or fill her head with doubts about what she's doing. I may suggest she ask her doctor certain questions, but why would I want to upset a woman who is in such a fragile state? And yet, if you're in the chat rooms, you're very likely to read upsetting comments, intended for someone else, but as frightening as if they were talking directly to you. It's as if a bunch of people are sitting around a campfire telling ghost stories that all involve you as the terrified coed who's being menaced by the crazed killer.

Realizing that chat rooms were toxic to me was probably the first inkling I had that I was not going to live up to the media-generated expectations of How We Do Breast Cancer. From the first visit until the last, my inner voice was shouting, "Danger! Get out!" but I ignored it, because I thought it must be wrong this time. I was too caught up in trying to follow the script. And I thought the script said you'll find wisdom and comfort in the chat rooms.

The Kingdom of the Well and the Kingdom of the Sick

Looking back on it, I think I was trying to fit in to the breast cancer community, but I just couldn't find my place. I was lost in the space between the two worlds Dr. Susan Love describes as the "temporarily immortal" versus "the world of the defectives."

Susan Sontag wrote in *Illness as Metaphor* that each of us holds dual citizenship, in the Kingdom of the Well and the Kingdom of the Sick.

I didn't feel as though I belonged to either kingdom. I clung fiercely to my home in the land of the healthy, and refused to believe residents who told me, gently, that I couldn't live in Healthyville anymore. It was shattering to my ego and my sense of self. I'd spent my whole life there; I had a great place, I knew where all the best shops and restaurants and schools were ... and I was happy in Healthyville. Couldn't I just get a short-term sublet in Breastcancerworld briefly and then move back into my old place when I'd finished treatment?

I could not imagine how I could possibly live in Breastcancerworld. But since it felt like the whole planet expected me to move there, I reluctantly gave it a try. I felt pressured to go meekly into the Pink Ghetto, but I couldn't stay there. I felt like an alien. I couldn't breathe, I couldn't find sustenance, I couldn't wait to get the hell out of there and back to Healthyville, even if I had to "pass" to blend back in with the locals there.

The point is, the pink bubble is not one size fits all. Don't assume that someone else's experience will be yours—or that you're doing it wrong if you reject the expectations of those around you.

What a relief it was when I finally understood that I had to avoid the chat rooms for my own sanity. It felt like a gift, and in a way it was; the gift of freedom to continue to be me, unchanged.

As I write this, I know how lucky I was that I wasn't forced to move full-time into Breastcancerworld. I pray that my luck holds. I will be so angry with the cosmos if I have a recurrence of breast cancer. Then, chat rooms, look out. I will become the message poster from Hell. But for now, the truth is, I'm not so much livin' large in Healthyville as I am hunkered down on the outskirts, living on the wrong side of the tracks. In my new and far less pleasant neighborhood:

I get stomach cancer a lot. Pretty much every time I eat raw vegetables. Luckily, it's cured by popping a TUMS. All the little moles and freckles I've had for years can be melanoma in the middle of the night, until my dermatologist tells me they're absolutely nothing. I don't want to be a hypochondriac, but the mind does go there sometimes.

Every six months, I have the heart-pounding, sweat-inducing nightmare of mammograms and sonograms, which too often turn up something that needs "further checking out" but so far have not found anything serious.

Speaking of sweat-inducing, the drug I take every day, tamoxifen, makes me sweaty. I'm always too hot, which is not the same as having hot flashes (I know from experience), but it is only marginally less embarrassing to be constantly flushed and damp than it is to have it come on with a dramatic and unexpected flourish. Half-moon-shaped sweat stains around your neckline look kind of great in the gym, but in the office? Not so much.

The bars here have a one-drink limit. If you're diligent about minimizing your risk of recurrence, you take seriously the findings that show a relationship between alcohol consumption and breast cancer. The same goes for soy products— bye bye, Boca Burgers, and sayonara, edamame. I loved you, but . . .

And then there are the obsessive self-exams. I'm like a

horny fifteen-year-old boy around my breasts, constantly feeling myself up. I search every square inch for lumps, which is ironic considering that I never felt my tumor when I actually had one, or the benign growth I had in the other breast the next year.

And yes, my part of Healthyville has an overabundance of plus-size stores for those of us who've become overabundant in the butts and thighs. I don't blame tamoxifen for the ten pounds I've gained but I do blame it for making it almost impossible to lose the weight. There is no scientific proof that tamoxifen or the other hormone therapy, the aromatase inhibitors like Arimidex, cause weight gain. But it is such a common, almost universal complaint about tamoxifen that I have to say, if it walks like a duck and it quacks like a duck, it's probably a woman on tamoxifen.

I feel the disapproval of many of you readers. After all, compared to what I could be suffering, what's so bad about a boozeless, fat, sweaty, hypochondriacal life? To thousands of women, that would be a huge improvement. I know that and I hope they'll join me here on the wrong side of the tracks in Healthyville very soon. I am describing how my life has changed, and not for the better, because this is a way of acknowledging what others may also be experiencing. And also because I'd rather laugh about it than complain about it.

A Lesson Not Learned from Breast Cancer

"Don't be too hard on yourself. Especially those of us who are type A women, take-charge people. I beat myself up because I wanted to go back to being able to do everything. I got mad at myself.

"We're always waiting for breast cancer to 'teach' us something. But it really just gave me an opportunity to listen to what my brain already knew—that you can plan everything and something will screw it up, so just go with it and don't think you can be in control of everything."

—Courtney Bugler, writer, blogger

Part Two

OUR BODIES, BUT NOT OUR SELVES

Chapter Four

It's Not About the ~~Bike~~ Breast

When you have breast cancer, the first question a lot of people ask is some variation of, "What are they going to do to you?" And by that I had the clear impression they meant, How much surgery are you going to need?

Everybody assumes that you're going to live, it's just a question of what you're going to look like in a low-cut dress.

The assumption in our breast-obsessed society seems to be that nothing could be more shattering to a woman than a mastectomy. After all, our very femaleness is at stake, isn't it?

Or is it?

I mean, obviously, a diagnosis of breast cancer is devastating—any potentially fatal medical condition whose treatment involves amputating a part of our bodies is horrific. Remembering how angry and violated I felt after my lumpectomy, I can only imagine how much worse it would have been if my whole breast had been removed.

But not necessarily because the amputated part was a breast. I can't say it would be more painful to lose a breast than any other body part. I would hate to lose anything, except the loose bit of skin on my neck that makes me look like a turkey.

Breast cancer for me was never an assault on my femininity; it was an assault on my personhood. Besides, it was only a temporary attack, unlike some of the real assaults on my femininity that I've been dealing with for years. If you're over forty, you know what I'm talking about. Random chin hairs, brittle bones, wrinkles, gray hair, and worst of all, that damned Cloak of Invisibility that falls over us when we enter a room full of younger women. Tits or no tits, you could be naked and nobody would notice you.

Although I never thought about it much until I had a lumpectomy, I realize now that I'm not one of those women who considers her breasts to be the home office of her Womanhood. My femininity doesn't reside in any one place; it is me, the whole me-ness of me, and can't be sliced off in pieces.

(And yes, I do know something about having random female body parts surgically removed. When I had a partial hysterectomy years ago a number of people asked me if I felt less like a woman afterward. I felt less like talking to them, but no, I didn't feel less like a woman.)

As for my breasts, I was never one to focus too much attention on them. They were just sort of there, where they were supposed to be, neither too big nor too small. If my body were a neighborhood, my breasts were the quiet, pleasant, clean-cut folks who lived next door and kept to themselves.

("I don't understand it," my stunned thighs would say on the local news after my lumpectomy, "those breasts never gave anybody any trouble before this.") They looked nice in sweaters and low-cut tops, and once the braless look came in they were happy to bounce around. I was unself-conscious about them.

That was the relationship then, and pretty much that's the relationship now. In my world of body-image issues, unself-conscious is tantamount to self-worship.

My husband, Dennis, on the other hand, would miss my breasts very, very much. He is a breast man in general, and a *my* breast man in particular. He's an artist who has painted my breasts many times. Sometimes when he expresses his affection for them, in the grabby, enthusiastic ways that guys do, it makes me uncomfortable. I can't help but worry how he would be affected if I had a recurrence or a new cancer that resulted in mastectomy. I'm afraid he would be sadder even than I would be. He says he would just deal with it, and he would, and I'm sure he'd be very grateful that the surgery had saved my life, but I fear that subconsciously he'd be deeply disappointed at having to live out his life with a breastless, or reconstructed, wife.

And although I would understand his reaction, it would piss me off.

One of the things I hate most about breast cancer is that it has made me nervous about how much my husband loves my breasts.

What kind of a world is it where a guy says, "Hey, baby,

nice rack," and the first thing you can think of is, "Yeah . . . for now"?

"Sin Tetas No Hay Paraiso," or, "Without Tits There Is No Paradise."

I had never seen the word *"tetas"* before a story in *Variety* about this hit television show in Colombia that has been picked up for development by NBC, but I immediately added *"tetas"* to the seemingly endless list of terms used for breasts. A short sampling, courtesy of many sources, would include:

Boobs, boobies, bosoms, hooters, tits, titties, tetas, knockers, headlights, head lamps, love lamps, high beams, devil's dumplings, sweater puppets, sweater muffins, sweater puppies, fun bags, chesticles, breasticles, tatas, the rack, the girls, the twins, B1 and B2, badoinkies, bazoombas, Ben and Jerry, Bert and Ernie, Bonnie and Clyde, Fred and Ethel, melons, cantaloupes, cassavas, mangoes, honeydews, twin peaks, chimichangas, coconuts, pumpkins, jugs, pointer sisters, flap doodles, Betty and Veronica, Betty and Wilma, Thelma and Louise, boom boom rockets, glad bags, girlie guns, golden globes, grapefruits, lady lumps, lady humps, milk duds, milk jugs, milk bombs, nay nays, norks, Nefertitties, and Tora Boras.

And if you think those nicknames are creative, take a look at this list of objects inserted into breasts over the years.

Things Women Have Implanted in Their Breasts to Make Them Appear Bigger

- Fat transplants from bellies, backs, and bottoms (1890s, 1930s–'40s) Result: Fat reabsorbed, left unsightly lumps
- Paraffin injections (1890s–1920s)
  Result: Horrendous lumps, a.k.a. "wax cancer"
- Liquid silicone injections (1940s until banned in the United States in 1965)
  Result: gangrene, infections, other complications sometimes requiring mastectomy
- Glass balls, ivory, rubber, wool, ox cartilage (1950s)
  Result: What do you think?
- Sponges (1950s)
  Result: Led to infections, disfigurement
- Silicone, saline implants (1962 to present)
  Result: Safe, we think

I'm not sure what the thought process is for a woman who says to her doctor, "Okay, yes, go ahead and implant some glass balls in my breasts. I'm sure they'll look and feel very natural."

Yet, there were women in the early to mid 1900s who said, "Bring 'em on," or whatever ladies said back then, to glass-ball breast implants, ox-cartilage breast implants, wool implants, ivory, and more.

Ouch.

No wonder the '20s roared.

Given the century-old impulse to implant, you may not be surprised to learn that federal law requires insurance companies to pay for reconstructive surgery after mastectomies. It's called the Women's Health and Cancer Rights Act of 1998. It not only mandates coverage for reconstruction, but also requires reimbursement for plastic surgery on the other breast, too, if desired, to make them a matched set. And there's no statute of limitations on it; a woman can decide years after a mastectomy that she wants a reconstructed breast.

Insurance also covers the cost of the best prosthetic boobs money can buy, for women who don't want reconstruction.

God Bless America, where breasts are a federally mandated entitlement.

Most women who have mastectomies elect to have reconstructive surgery, either immediately or after they've completed cancer treatment. I have no proof, but I would guess that the fact that breasts can be reconstructed gives many women the courage to get regular mammograms and to go to their doctors when they feel something unusual. I never thought about implants as lifesavers, (let alone afterlife savers, as in Colombia), but maybe they are.

I do know a lot of women who are thrilled to have them.

Vivian McDevitt, who is forty-seven years old, was told by three doctors (she got a second and a third opinion) that she needed a mastectomy; ultimately, she decided to have the nondiseased breast removed as well. She is a wife, mother, and working woman, and has one of the most positive attitudes I've ever encountered. That applied to her surgery and reconstruction.

"Your breasts do not define whether you are female or not," she told me. "If you want to talk about sexuality, it does affect that, because you don't feel your nipples anymore. So there is a certain sadness. But I got a flat belly out of it and I would make the same decision if I had to do it all over again."

Vivian's reconstruction involved taking flesh from her tummy to fashion breast replacement tissue. She also was happy to go from very large breasts to a much more manageable size. And she likes the way she looks now, in clothes and in a bathing suit.

What about the women who decide not to have reconstructed breasts, and not to wear fake ones, either? I've talked to several who say that they felt they had to explain, and justify, their decisions over and over. They reported that the pressure to do something to fill in their chests was not always subtle. It's also not new.

Twenty years ago the lesbian feminist African-American poet Audre Lorde wrote about being told to wear a prosthetic breast when she visited her doctor because, the nurses said, it was "bad for morale" in the office when she showed up without it. We may have progressed past that kind of blatant insensitivity, but the pressure to blend back into society and be invisible as a breast cancer survivor frustrated Lorde and many women who have their own reasons for rejecting reconstruction or prostheses.

Audre Lorde would have loved the artist and designer Jacqueline Skaggs. Jacqueline chose not to have breast reconstruction because it just wasn't necessary for her. As she put it, "I don't know how many times I've said, 'This wasn't a political decision, a statement maker.' The decision to walk the earth without a fake breast was a simple one based on my own personal ideologies and tolerances."

Jacqueline objects to the idea that moving on with your life without a reconstruction or a prosthetic breast is somehow the "wrong" decision, but she was frustrated by the lack of stylish clothing for women whose chests were asymmetrical.

So she started a line of clothing and jewelry called Rhea Belle for women who have had mastectomies and plan to live their lives without fake breasts of any kind. Her clothes are designed to allow women to "embrace their natural architecture."

I asked her how her husband felt about her decision. She smiled and shrugged a little.

"He said, 'It's your body. I just want you healthy.' I was glad, but his attitude wasn't a factor in my decision," she told me.

The blogger and University of British Columbia professor Mary Bryson had a simple attitude about mastectomy.

"It's a very individualized decision," she told me. "A lot of the medical thinking about breast cancer is driven by 'save the breast' logic over 'save the life.' My primary goal was not to save my breast. I haven't ever been particularly attached to my breasts, whereas I'm very attached to my life."

Mary identifies herself as "queer"; and her attitudes about her body and her self-image are different.

"It's some indication of the general social stigma attached to being breastless that it's always considered a tragedy that must be corrected. I went through a great deal of sadness before the surgery. I cried every day. I was very, very sad about having to undergo an amputation. Mastectomy is a violent, significant, highly visible, not very sophisticated surgery. It was a violation of the integrity of my body."

As Mary wrote in a blog post called "What Am I Missing?":

I think that people should be totally supported to seek out whatever brings them peace and happiness following the removal of one or both breasts. I am happy that a whack of tax dollars are going to pay for breast reconstruction for women undergoing mastectomies. What irks me is that my own choice to go breastless, and keep it that way, is not being supported.

I have to say I don't think I could put the "me" in mastectomy by forgoing breast reconstruction. If my goal was, and would always be, to minimize breast cancer's impact

on my life, how could 1 leave untouched a crater literally
made by cancer's violent impact on my body? I think I'd
want to rebuild that area as soon as possible. I understand
the argument that by blending back in, looking as normal
as possible, we "reinforce our own isolation and invisibility
from each other, as well as the false complacency of a society which would rather not face the results of its own in-
sanities," as Audre Lorde wrote in *The Cancer Journals*.

I respect that point of view, but it's not my point of
view.

Self-Esteem, or Just Self, Steamed?

Of all the well-meaning but thoughtless things that people
say to women with breast cancer, near the top of my list is
telling a woman who's facing a mastectomy not to worry,
because she can have reconstructed boobs that are perkier
and nicer than her real ones. You don't have to be political
to find that notion really annoying. People who tell you
you'll be better than ever very likely have no idea how
much extra surgery, pain, and potential problems reconstruction can mean. Or that the new breasts, while high
and firm, do not include your real nipples, in the vast majority of cases. If someone cheerfully tells you that you can
get a new breast that's even better than the one that the
doctors will slice off (and this happens to women facing

surgery all the time), I suggest you reply: "Really? Can I pick out a part of *your* body that might be improved by cutting it off and replacing it with a perky replica?"

I think what it comes down to is an effort to pull you over to the emotional safety of the Bright Side (for them).

They want to believe that a reconstructed breast will fix you right up, and if you don't agree, maybe there's something wrong with your head. Call the attitude police, quick.

What they may not understand is not just that breast cancer has left an enduring scar (whether you have reconstruction or not), but that there's no GPS system for helping to get you through the tunnel of grief and anger and out to acceptance. There's no official mourning period for a lost breast, no calendar that tells you where you are in your process. You can't rush it, and you can't be rushed by friends and family who expected, or hoped, that when you finished the treatment process, you'd be "over it" and back to your old self.

It takes time to adjust to your new body, inside and out.

I got away relatively unscathed, and that's partly why I was able to accept the damage done to my body pretty easily. I still had two breasts, after all. But I also believe that the fact that I wasn't exactly in love with my body in the first place helped me a lot. In this case, it was better not to have loved and lost than never to have loved at all. If nothing else, I already knew what it felt like to be disappointed by my body. Every. Damned. Day. Having a run-in with breast cancer didn't change that.

You see, on my breast cancer "journey," I couldn't find a single sign that read THIS WAY TO BODY ACCEPTANCE. Somewhere around the time that I admitted to myself how elated I was to be losing weight during chemo, I also realized that while breast cancer can be a temporary problem, body-image issues are forever. That is why the regular weigh-in at the doctor's office during chemotherapy was definitely the high point of chemo days for me. Early on, Dr. Chuang expressed concern and told me I would have to be careful not to lose too much weight. I remember that I nodded compliantly but thought, *Yeah, right. Like that's gonna happen.* I also remember feeling a little guilty for fooling my doctor, as if I were being caught with my hand outside the cookie jar.

Concerns about weight gain are extremely common, by the way. Dr. Bonni Gearhart believes it's easy to understand why.

"Weight gain is the biggest issue for my patients. It happens to some because they eat comfort food, some of them are depressed, most of them stop going to the gym and stop exercising altogether during chemo."

"Does all that focus on our weight mean we're hopelessly shallow?" I asked.

"I don't think it's shallow at all," she replied emphatically. "You can't look at the constant media images of women or live in the corporate world and then tell us we're shallow when you cut off our breasts and our hair falls out."

Yeah! What she said. On the other hand, if you're afraid you're developing a dependency on macaroni and cheese, you may be able to consult with a nutritionist through your doctor's practice.

I suppose my endless, big-caboose-induced self-esteem issues, unstoppable even by cancer, make me a feminist's nightmare, a poster child for that whole, crushed-by-the-patriarchy-over-unattainable-beauty thing. It was one of those problems I had hoped breast cancer would fix. But since breast cancer doesn't fix anything, much less a lifetime of slavishly trying to conform to the Evil Corporate Patriarchy's ideal of beauty, it didn't happen.

Breast cancer didn't change those concerns; it only confirmed that the way I evaluate my appearance is through a fat filter. If I were to lose a breast altogether someday, I suspect it would only intensify my desire to be slim, to control the aspects of my body that I *can* (sort of) control.

It seems kind of nuts to think that just because you'd had a disease, you'd suddenly be able to erase a lifetime of thinking one way about yourself and replace it with the opposite way. Maybe if they made ribbons and bracelets for women who hate their big butts, as a reminder that we should love ourselves, I'd feel differently. What color is the ribbon for Cellulite Awareness, anyway?

The real issue here is not whether I can be happy with a life of self-denial or guilt every time a piece of cake calls out to me. It's whether I can feel desirable and worthy of love in whatever shape I'm in—fat, thin, with breasts or without. I try to remember that it's ridiculous to hold myself to higher standards for lovability than the people who already love me do.

Too bad there isn't a chemotherapy for body-image neuroses. I would happily take it, especially if it was chocolate-flavored.

A Lesson Not Learned from Breast Cancer

"I was always a fighter; I have been my whole life. I inherited mental toughness from my father, who was an aggressive thinker, spunky and assertive. I knew going into it that I would beat breast cancer, even if I haven't totally done it yet. With all I've been through, I'm still an optimist. I always knew I had it in me to get through tough things, but this has been ridiculous!"

—Theresa Flais

Chapter Five

Help Them
Help You

Lesson Four:

Never be afraid to admit that
you need help. It's a sign of
strength, not weakness.

I would say that the single most important lesson I have learned in my life is that there's no reason to be ashamed to ask for help when you need it. If it's a question of muddling through alone and doing a mediocre job, or asking for help so that you can do a great job, it's pretty obvious what the right choice is. It doesn't make you a burden.

When you're dealing with breast cancer, the odds are very, very good that you're going to need some help. Ask for it.

Besides, whatever the crisis, everybody *wants* to help— they get to be heroes, after all, when they ride in on a white horse to save the day.

From the Shadows to the Spotlight

Of course, if you want help, you have to acknowledge that you have a problem, like, say, fatigue and nausea brought on by cancer treatment. It's hard to believe, but until the mid-'70s, it was almost never talked about in public. In fact, forty years ago, doctors didn't even tell their patients they had breast cancer. (They'd talk about lumps and masses, as if the women didn't know what they meant.) Fortunately, thanks to the Breast Cancer Awareness campaign and the very vocal advocates for the disease, nowadays we think nothing of talking about it publicly.

One of the first prominent women to disclose that she had breast cancer was then—First Lady Betty Ford, in 1974. Just a few weeks after her husband, Gerald Ford, pardoned Richard Nixon, she announced that she had breast cancer and would undergo a radical mastectomy. A few weeks after that, the vice president's wife, Happy Rockefeller, discovered that she, too, had breast cancer.

There was no twenty-four-hour cable back then, of course, so to say that their breast cancers received massive media coverage is an overstatement compared to, say, Paris Hilton's limo ride from her parents' house to the county jail. But still, Ford and Rockefeller did bring breast cancer front and center into the national conversation, prompting lots of magazine articles (in newsmagazines, not just the women's pages) and television stories.

Mrs. Ford was remarkably open about her experience. She used her breast cancer diagnosis as an opportunity to prove to millions of Americans that the disease is not an automatic death sentence. After her surgery, there was even a photo of her in the hospital, tossing a football to her husband. (Which must have hurt like hell, given that she had a radical mastectomy, a procedure that removes muscle and lymph nodes and leaves most women permanently debilitated.)

These days, you can't pick up a women's magazine without reading some woman's personal story about breast cancer, so much so that when I called to tell a Hollywood-based colleague about my diagnosis, he joked, "My, aren't we trendy."

It was just my luck that the one time in the entire breast cancer process that I was keenly aware of how desperately I needed help, and asked everybody for it, was a time when I got no help at all. It involved making a decision about what form of chemotherapy to have. Thank goodness there was a clearheaded seventeen-year-old around to consult.

My Chemical Romance

About a week after surgery (although it felt like a month), Dr. Simmons called me with the results of the pathology tests on the tumor she'd removed. It was almost all good news, relatively speaking, of course. The tumor was small, there were no lymph nodes involved, and no cancer cells in my bone marrow (she takes a little sample from her patients' hip bones while they're under anesthesia). The tumor was estrogen positive, which is good, because it's easier to treat, and HER-2 negative, which means the tumor wasn't producing an abundance of a protein that would transmit a message to stimulate the production of cancer cells. Dr. Simmons sounded super-optimistic, so I was relieved, of course.

Except that they still wanted me to do chemotherapy. Now that I was doing my research and beginning to understand the ramifications of chemo on my body, I didn't like what I was learning. One kind of chemo caused heart problems in some (a few) women. Another kind had the possibility of causing leukemia. This was terrifying to me. Breast cancer was all soft and pink and you could walk for the cure, but leukemia? Leukemia seemed like I would be trading up on the serious life-threatening cancer scale.

And then there was chemo brain. In 2004 doctors were beginning to acknowledge that for a fair number of women, chemotherapy causes cognitive loss, maybe permanently. Cognitive loss, it seemed to me, was another way of saying "brain damage." Women who have chemo brain report an inability to concentrate, to remember certain words, and to handle more than one task at a time.

Now, all of these possible side effects are bad enough when you really, truly, definitely need chemotherapy to be sure your cancer is gone. In my case, I was being told to do chemo even though at best it would increase the odds of avoiding a recurrence by no more than three percentage points. And, as Dr. Chuang explained to me, when you consider that the risk factor of causing leukemia or heart damage is about 1 percent, the potential benefit of doing chemo seemed to me to be marginal at best.

There was one factor weighing in favor of chemo—because although it was a "good news" tumor in most respects, it did have one bad-ass characteristic. It was what is known as a Grade 3 tumor, the most aggressive grade. Dr. Chuang said she'd have chemo if she were in my situation, and Dr. Simmons had been recommending it from the beginning. It was weird how I feared chemo so much more than I feared cancer, but that's the way it was. Still, I went for it, and this was my reasoning:

With chemo added to the mix of other treatments (surgery, radiation, and tamoxifen), I got to decrease my risk of recurrence by about three percentage points.

I pictured myself in a room with ninety-nine other women who had had breast cancer. A guy in a white coat with a clipboard comes in and says, "Okay, ninety-seven of you get to leave this room now and you'll never have cancer again. Uh, not so fast, Shelley. Where do you think you're going? Go stand next to those other two women. Sorry about this, ladies. But you didn't think doing chemo was worth that extra two or three percentage points, remember?"

I didn't want to be left behind with the other two ladies in the cancer clubhouse.

My inner voice was saying, "You'll hate yourself if you didn't do every single thing you could and you have a recurrence." Which was true, and frankly, I try very hard never to get mad at me. I say the worst things to myself.

So I said yes to chemo. There was just one problem. I had to decide between two different but equally gross flavors of chemotherapy.

I truly didn't want either, but I was offered the choice of doing the ugly, AC/T variety (adriamycin, cytoxan, and then taxol), which meant four months of harsh treatment and baldness but then it was over, or a slightly milder, much slower chemotherapy called CMF (cytoxan, methotrexate, and fluorouracil), which would leave me a lot of my hair but take six long months and many more visits to the chemo lab. Either would be appropriate for me, I was told.

Dr. Chuang left it entirely up to me. And I simply couldn't make up my mind between two lousy choices. My daughter, Julia, summed it up perfectly.

"Wow, Mom, you have to choose between your two worst personality traits," she observed, "impatience and vanity."

She was exactly right. On the one hand, I did want to get it over with as quickly as possible, and suffer with many fewer needles, but on the other hand, I envisioned myself working throughout, and I didn't want to be bald and look sickly. As far as potential serious risks, they were both scary, but AC/T seemed slightly more toxic to me. I was simply incapable of choosing a course of action. I asked my sister Lisa what she would do, and after doing research (she is a Ph.D. in anthropology and understands science far better than I), she weighed in with an opinion based on potential risks and long-term side effects. So did several other people. Nobody's opinions mattered, though.

You know how when someone gives you a piece of advice and it just clicks with you, you suddenly feel so relieved, because you've finally heard exactly what you needed to hear?

Well, that never happened in this case. Everybody whose opinion I sought gave me a clear and rational answer. I talked with my friend Rachel Bellow about it repeatedly. We'd come to one conclusion, and then ten minutes later I'd have wandered off in the other direction.

Honestly, I had never in my life had such a difficult time making a decision.

Finally, at the hair salon, I told my stylist that I was leaning toward doing it the quicker way, and that I was going to have to get a wig.

"No problem. Bring it in and we'll cut it and style it. We've done it for lots of clients. Don't worry, it'll look great," she said cheerfully. I asked her for the name of the best wig store in town, and she gave me two choices that she said had excellent selections.

It was at that very moment that my inner voice, which had apparently been on vacation, came back to work.

"No fucking way," it said softly. There were tears in my eyes.

And then I knew. It was vanity over impatience for me.

I kept my hair (mostly), I kept my eyebrows, and I kept having to go for a seemingly endless set of chemo sessions.

And after every single chemo treatment, I went to work, just as I had wanted to do.

Working Girls (with Breast Cancer)

I didn't tell everyone at my workplace about it. It wasn't that I was embarrassed or ashamed of it; I just didn't want everybody to treat me differently than they normally would. And I was at work instead of at home specifically to get my mind off breast cancer; I didn't want to talk about it all day long.

One of the first people I told at Air America was my dear friend and co–programming executive, the hilarious comedian and producer Lizz Winstead. I told her that it wasn't a secret, exactly, but that I wanted to be the one to tell people, and I'd do it when it felt like the right time. Of course she agreed.

Hours later I noticed Rachel Maddow, one of Lizz's on-air cohosts, was treating me with unusual attention and courtesy. She breezed into my office for a chat, eventually asking me if I wanted her to get me some lunch. When I said no, I'd go out myself, she insisted on keeping me company. We'd never once had lunch together before. I wasn't even sure she liked me, to tell you the truth. (We became very good friends.) Yet there she was, hanging on my every word, and while none of those words was "cancer," I just knew she knew.

"You told Rachel, didn't you?" I asked Lizz as soon as I saw her.

"I had to," she said. "I was afraid I might get all weird during the show and it could throw her off. This isn't just about you, you know," she said and laughed.

It never is. A big illness is about all the people affected by it, and most of us do have a circle of friends and family who worry and want to do something to help.

And if you work, as most of us do, it's pretty hard to keep it on the down low. Consider this scenario:

You're riding in an elevator at work and a male colleague steps in.

"Wow, your hair looks great," he exclaims.

"Thanks," you say crisply, hoping that's the end of it.

"Did you do something different?" he persists.

Hmmmm... how to reply?

"Why, yes, I did do something different. I'm having chemo for breast cancer and all my hair has fallen out, so this is actually a wig. I'm so glad you like it!"

This approach amounts to telling him:

"Jerkville City Limits. Population: You."

Perfect response if he happens to be a guy you need to get even with for something; otherwise, perhaps a tad harsh.

*Another choice might be to smile and quickly change
the subject. But then you've handed him a ticking time
bomb that will eventually become the Exploding Cancer
Gaffe, showering him with the shrapnel of disfiguring
embarrassment when he discovers the truth about your
groovy new 'do.*

*You have about three seconds to decide which one of
you is about to feel awful. Ready? Go.*

Okay, stop. There is no correct answer, only the one
that feels right at the moment. How you choose to handle
the "gee your hair looks terrific" moment depends on a lot
of factors, including your mood, your strength, and your
sense of security at work.

Just know that it's all part of the Working Girl's Guide
to Awkward Moments You Didn't See Coming When You
Got Breast Cancer. There will certainly be others—urgent
"excuse mes" shouted over your shoulder when you dash
off to the ladies' room as one or both ends of your digestive
tract threatens to erupt, say, or getting all sweaty during a
conversation with your boss, who knows what you're going
through, but probably still thinks you're perspiring because
you feel guilty about screwing something up. Or waking
up from a "quick" nap on the sofa in the ladies' lounge to
find a colleague tiptoeing past you, and realizing that probably half a dozen women have seen you passed out with
your mouth open for the entire duration of the lunch hour.

And, if you're wondering, yes, all of the above happened

to me at one point or another, except the wig thing, which happened to an executive who was still trying at that point in her treatment to "pass."

The people I was close to knew everything I was going through and helped me a lot. On chemo treatment days, I would try to get my work done before the drugs started to make me feel lousy, and that meant other people had to rearrange their schedules and sometimes scramble to finish their work earlier so I could sign off on it before leaving in mid-afternoon. (As with recreational drugs, when it came to chemo, timing was everything. I wanted to stay at work as long as I felt well enough, but if I waited too long, the drugs kicked in on the trip home, and that was a huge bummer, as we used to say.)

I didn't like having to inconvenience other people to accommodate my situation, but it was what I found I had to do. As time went on and the cumulative effects of months of chemo took their toll on my body, I continued to go to work every day, but I knew I was accomplishing less, and needing to ask for help more often.

This was all happening in the weeks leading up to election day, a very big event at the network, as you can imagine, and I had no intention of missing it. We did a special live campaign show every Sunday for the last several weeks before election day, and normally I would have gone in to make sure everything went well. But not in 2004. I needed to rest up on the weekends, and I had to delegate to other people some of the work I would normally have happily done myself. I didn't always ask for help explicitly, but I let help happen.

Far be it from me to tell any woman how to handle her breast cancer treatment, but I would like to share with you the experiences and wisdom of some other working women.

Theresa Flais is an amazing woman. A single mother of two boys living in Columbus, Ohio, she discovered at thirty-seven that she had breast cancer. Unfortunately, the initial diagnosis was way off—instead of needing a simple lumpectomy for an early-stage cancer, the doctors found advanced breast cancer. She ended up having a double mastectomy. Her mother was with her for some of her treatment, but she did much of it on her own.

"I had lots of offers of help, from neighbors and friends, and I always said no," she told me.

"That's just me. I didn't want to feel that I was burdening other people. It helped me get through it to do it all myself. But right after my mom left I got bronchitis and ended up going to the hospital. I actually drove myself to the hospital. I definitely should have asked for help then. That was pretty stupid. When I got back home, I did ask a neighbor to watch the boys for me. I see it more now than when I was in the situation, that I didn't want people to think I was sick . . . because then I would feel sicker."

Theresa is a theater director at a dinner theater in Columbus, and they were in the middle of rehearsals for a new production when she started chemo. She made it to the theater every day, because "it was an escape for me."

She went to chemo by herself "many times, until my church found out about me. They were shocked. Then they'd send someone to sit with me, people I didn't even know. As much as I appreciated it, after a while I felt like I had to entertain them! It's not my personality to let someone sit there feeling uncomfortable. Many of them are my dear friends now, but I've never told them that."

Theresa perhaps took too seriously the old adage "The show must go on." I think when the stage is a chemo suite, you're allowed to cancel a performance or two.

Anybody who makes decisions sometimes makes mistakes, and if you're going through breast cancer treatment you will have to make a lot of decisions, so you're bound to make some mistakes. Believe it or not, you do have a margin of error.

When the artist and designer Jacqueline Skaggs had breast cancer in 2001 she was working at a Baltimore museum. She had a lumpectomy and radiation, and she told almost no one at the museum. She didn't want to be treated differently by her coworkers, she says.

"In hindsight, I regret that decision," she told me. "It maintained a kind of segregation between the well and the sick, especially among women. But it was like I had blinders on. I was emotional and angry and I just wanted to get through it and survive."

Before her first surgery, Jacqueline's doctor told her, "If you need to have a mastectomy, you'll get an implant. No woman leaves my operating room without reconstruction."

Now that's a hell of a statement, isn't it? In its way, it is every bit as disempowering, and condescending, as in the bad old days when a woman suspected of breast cancer was expected to go meekly along with whatever her doctor did, and keep her opinions to herself. Jacqueline says she stayed with that doctor, though, because, other than the implant remark, which she hated, she was collaborative and respectful. She particularly liked that the doctor drew lots of diagrams and discussed her options with her as they went over her films together.

When the cancer returned in 2004, Jacqueline had moved to New York with her husband. This time there was no question that she would require a mastectomy, but this time, no doctor told her she would "need" an implant, and she opted not to have one. And this time, she talked to more people about what she was going through.

"The second time, I was much more open about it. I wanted to explore the reality of what I was experiencing with the people I love. Separating myself from my own group felt wrong."

An enormous part of Jacqueline's help came from Memorial Sloan-Kettering, through a program that pays all medical costs for some financially needy patients who qualify. She was unemployed at the time and had no insurance.

Without the help from Sloan-Kettering, it's hard to imagine how she would have paid for the medical treatment she needed to live.

Governor Jodi Rell made a point of being back on the job not two weeks after her mastectomy. Connecticut had watched another of its governors, Ella Grasso, struggle with ovarian cancer, which ultimately forced her to resign her office; she died just months later. Rell wanted everybody to know she, and their state, would be just fine. But she was wise enough to know her limits in the weeks following her surgery.

"I had to count on other people to help me," she told me. "I spent a lot of time at home in sweatpants. I did budgets from there, at the governor's mansion. I was a little embarrassed—I felt kind of sloppy. I finally told everyone working with me there to stop dressing up, get comfortable. One lesson I had really learned from years of experience, is you have to grow up and admit, 'You know what? I can't do everything. But I can be in charge and be satisfied.' "

I know that many women feel they have to tough it out as much as possible at work because of fear. They worry they'd lose their jobs or be penalized financially if they took too much time off or asked to work shorter days.

In fact, you may have rights under the Americans with Disabilities Act. If you need time off from work for treatment, or if you need to rest at work, you have the legal right to do so. You do not have to put up with discrimination.

If you're a business or professional woman in a leadership role, you do have to feel your way through the question of how much to reveal and share with your staff and coworkers. Obviously, Governor Rell was comfortable sharing a lot. But one thing she had to consider, as all executive women do, was how her cancer treatment affected the workplace and how that made her feel.

Amy Entelis, a senior vice president at ABC News, found out she had breast cancer just weeks after Peter Jennings revealed that he had lung cancer. The news division was still reeling from Peter's news; Amy didn't want to further complicate matters by announcing that she, too, had cancer. She told almost nobody at the network for quite a while, but she did call some friends who'd had breast cancer, including me. She had listened to my treatment story from beginning to end, and she called to ask me questions she didn't want to research herself.

We all have a limit to how much information we can take in. (Amy had also scared herself by spending too much time in chat rooms reading horror stories that were not her story. She reminded me recently that I told her to stay the hell out of chat rooms, a piece of advice she has passed along herself.)

Early in my own treatment, I stumbled across a kind of survivo-meter program at a very reputable Web site. It could tell you what your prognosis was. I carefully filled in all the pertinent information about my cancer, but at the last minute, I chickened out and didn't click "send." I just knew that I couldn't handle it if it gave me anything less than about a 98 percent chance of five-year survival.

The True Weapon of Mass Destruction

Those who describe chemotherapy as a kind of chemical warfare are either cancer patients or good students of history. The first chemotherapy drug was based on deadly mustard gas, which was used as a weapon in World War I. During World War II, after noting that some people accidentally exposed to mustard gas had very low white blood cell counts as a result, researchers thought it might work on lymphoma patients, whose bodies make too many white blood cells. They gave an injectable form of mustard gas to some lymphoma patients, who got better, temporarily. They were on the right track, anyway.

So you could say that mustard gas was the mother of all Weapons of *Mass* Destruction, if you're talking about tumor masses.

My Chemo Emo

I'm firmly committed to asking for help when I need it; sometimes it just takes me awhile to notice. Chemo was new to me and I didn't want to believe that it would knock me on my butt.

Chemotherapy, it must be remembered, is completely unnatural and counterintuitive. You've had surgery, you're just feeling good again, and then you let people deliberately make you sick by pouring poison into your body. In my case, I took pills for fourteen days each month; on the first and eighth day I also went in to the Chemo Cafe for an intravenous infusion of additional drugs. It began with an IV of saline, mixed with an antinausea drug, and when that was finished, the nurse would come in and pump a big honking syringe full of toxic "medicine" into a vein in my left hand.

The morning of my first chemo treatment, which occurred the very next day after we'd returned from Italy, I woke up gasping for air as these words became my first conscious thought:

I had cancer. Cancer.

Honestly, it was the first time I really, truly got it. I guess there's nothing like the prospect of big needles dumping poison into your veins to clarify the mind.

I wanted to talk about it with my husband, Dennis, still sleeping peacefully next to me. I rolled over and stared at him.

How the hell can he sleep like that? I would be wide awake if it were *me* taking *him* to his first chemo.

I can't be certain, but it may be that I gently nudged him with my foot, or possibly jabbed an elbow into his ribs, until he woke up. We got married in 1980, and had been through everything, richer and poorer, some sickness, mostly health, together. But we are very different kinds of people. He can sleep through a baby crying, a teenager out well past curfew, a financial crisis. I specialize in glaring at him and steaming over why he's unconscious and I have to do the worrying for both of us.

This was not going to be one of those times.

"Wake up. I have to have chemo today," I told him. "I had cancer."

"Yeah, I've heard that," he said.

We had an early-morning appointment, and in the car we listened to Air America. The morning show was always very funny, and it distracted me for a while.

By the time we got up to the doctor's office I was in a controlled panic, which means I look calm on the outside but I'm mentally stripping off all my clothes and running naked down the street screaming, "Help!"

The chemo room smelled of floor polish; it's an odor that can cause me to gag to this day when I smell it. There were no other patients there. A very nice nurse greeted us and sat me down in the first white leather lounge chair.

Dennis paid attention and asked questions when things didn't seem right to him.

Once the needle was inserted, it wasn't so bad. (Or so I told myself, still the reigning Queen of Denial.) The nurse was extremely caring, and because it was a quick infusion treatment, rather than a slow drip that can take hours, the whole procedure was relatively fast—about a half hour all told.

I decided that the next time, one week later, I could go alone. This, I believe, was only partly due to my ongoing denial. It was also prompted by the need to prove to myself and everybody around me how tough I was.

What a big mistake. I wasn't all that tough. The second chemo treatment was much harder for me. For one thing, without having someone there to impress with my bravery, I could really feel how much the damned needle hurt. For another, I'd had a week's worth of toxic slime in my system at that point, and I was starting to feel it. But the worst part was not having anyone there just to keep me distracted while I was hooked up to the poison machine. My self-confidence dissolved with every drip, and when the IV machine began flashing a warning about its line being clogged, I had visions of a killer gob of goo coursing straight into my brain.

("Poor Shelley. If only someone had been there to fetch the nurse before her head exploded all over everything, she would have lived to a ripe old age. But no, she had to prove how tough she was.")

A few minutes later the nurse returned and, noticing

the warning signal, wheeled the machine over and casually pushed the reset button.

Potential bursting brain crisis averted.

Still, the whole experience unnerved me and I felt awful the rest of the day. I was convinced that I would have been in much better shape, both physically and emotionally, if I'd had someone with me. That evening I told my friend Rachel about it, and she volunteered to be my chemo buddy whenever I needed her. We had great conversations, she made me laugh a lot, and when things got nasty or especially painful she would just pull up a chair closer to me and hold my hand. My sister Lisa came in from Princeton at least once a month to be with me, which meant giving up a big chunk of her day. She would say helpful things like, "Okay, whatever you do, don't look at your hand," in the calmest voice imaginable, when there was blood dripping all over it from some kind of IV problem, and she shared my silent exasperation when the nurse had to do an inordinate amount of poking and jamming to get the needle into a vein. Best of all, she had an almost encyclopedic memory for the jokes I was missing from *The Daily Show*, since I couldn't stay awake for it while I was on chemo.

"Professional Martyr" was never on my list of booths to visit on Career Day in high school, and as the long months of chemo wore me down, I knew I needed to ask for help more frequently. I was neediest for the two weeks I was "on" chemo each month.

During those two weeks, I had no appetite at all. This was a very strange experience for someone who generally thinks about food almost all the time. There was just nothing at all that appealed to me, and while you might think that I, as a lifelong dieter, would find that to be kind of a silver lining in the chemo cloud, it was actually kind of unnerving, because I wasn't in charge of it. After a while I would test my loss of appetite by going into a bakery near my office and standing in front of a display case filled with cupcakes and scones and cookies, with the idea that I would have absolutely anything I wanted. Under normal circumstances I could eat my weight in chocolate cupcakes—too bad I can't be weighed in cupcake units, instead of pounds—but during chemo, nothing doing. I might as well have been standing in front of a case of frosted lawn clippings.

During the second two weeks of the month, when I was off chemo so my body could recover sufficiently to poison it some more, I was able to eat again, even if I didn't enjoy it much. There was a constant metallic taste in my mouth, a common side effect of one of the drugs I was taking, which distorted the flavor of virtually everything. My beloved morning coffee tasted brackish, gum was all wrong, and some of my regular comfort food favorites, like yogurt with fruit and granola, and matzo ball soup, were ruined for me for all time. I lost ten pounds, and yes, I considered that a good thing.

It didn't last, though—just as the bad taste in my mouth

eventually went away and the queasy stomach ultimately settled itself, so too did my weight return. Sadly, I had a local recurrence of big butt–itis.

I will spare you the descriptions of gastrointestinal issues of every kind you can imagine; suffice it to say that my body was in revolt and doing things that were revolting.

Helping You Help Her

You can see why I depended more and more on other people to give me a hand as time went on. A mistake people sometimes made with me, and that I have made when offering my help to others, is to ask, "Is there anything I can do to help you?" When you're feeling crappy and overwhelmed, that question may be too broad. You need help with *everything*, including deciding what you most need help with; you're too wiped out to play project manager for your own treatment. Now that I've been on both sides of that question, I think it's more helpful to make concrete offers that are specific.

Sometimes it's as simple as calling the person and asking if there's anything she feels like eating, and then bringing it to her. Or maybe it's walking her dog, especially at night (hey, you said you wanted to help). If she works, you could do the errands that she normally does on the weekends or evenings. Dry cleaning, groceries, schlepping her kids, making some dinner for her family, especially food that could go in the fridge or freezer for another day. Bringing over cookies or videos for her kids. Come on, people, you can figure this out.

And call her or e-mail her regularly to check in. It's amazing how much a quick phone call can do to restore spirits when they begin to flag. I had lots of phone calls and e-mails, but there were people who told my husband or daughter they were afraid to call because they feared they'd disturb me. I wish I had thought to put out an all-points e-mail to everybody at the beginning of the process, suggesting good times to call, but it didn't even occur to me. I just figured whenever people called, it would be fine, because I would be fine.

Yes, it was just another example of being too blasé and, frankly, completely clueless about how I would deal with chemo. Sometimes being in denial will come back to bite you in the bum.

Playing the Cancer Card

Promise me that if you have to go through cancer treatment, you will play the Cancer Card. Because sometimes, no matter how much you want to convince the world and yourself that you're self-sufficient, managing very well, doing just fine, you really need to play the Cancer Card. Shamelessly.

This is not exactly the same thing as asking for help. This is asking for special favors and treatment because you had (have) breast cancer. This is taking advantage of people, not because you "deserve it," but because you can. Here are some things you might want to try.

- Getting out of a speeding ticket. ("Sorry, Officer, I'm late to a chemotherapy session and I guess I was a little anxious to get there. You know, *to save my life*.")
- Ask your mother for a family heirloom that you know your sister also wants. ("Come on, Mom, give it to me first, and then she can have it after I die. It's a win-win.") Your mom and your sister will be too shocked and horrified to say no.
- Order a bunch of stuff for yourself on QVC, and when it comes and your husband freaks out, blame it on chemo brain.
- Refuse to change the kitty litter or walk the dog, because your immune system is compromised. ("Do you want me to end up in the hospital because I was exposed to deadly animal poop germs?")
- Use it to avoid being dragged into any kind of social obligation or extracurricular work event. The soap opera writer and blogger Courtney Bugler says not only does she play the card herself whenever she wants to duck an event, she encourages

her friends to use her as an excuse, too. ("I'd love
to come but my friend Courtney has breast cancer
and I have to go over and cook for her tonight.")

Letting your friend borrow your Cancer Card is the
height of generosity, don't you think?

I played the card only occasionally, which, looking back
on it, was a huge wasted opportunity. I got Dennis to walk
the dog every night, whether it was a chemo week or not. I
ducked a few social events, but mostly I had to prove to
myself and my family that I was okay, and didn't need special consideration. What was I thinking?

Even worse was the lackluster way I played the card at
work. I took no sick days, none, because I didn't want to go
home and obsess about the crap coursing through my veins.
(My friend David Bender, our political director, helpfully
suggested one day that I try to think of the pills I was taking as my friends, not as poison. That would have been a
good idea if the last two syllables of the pill's name weren't
pronounced "toxin," as in Cytoxan.)

It was important to me to stay distracted. Still, I could
definitely have complained more about how I felt in order
to get people to be more cooperative and not come in to
complain about petty crap. And it would have been so satis-
fying, when someone called in sick, to snicker at them and
say, "You're telling me that you're too sick to come to work?
Because *I'm* here . . . and I'm having chemo, you wuss!"

Believe me, I was very tempted to do that, but I resisted

the impulse to try to guilt an entire radio network. That was as close to noble as I ever got; I wanted to lead by example.

The fact that no one was paying attention to my nobility made it all kind of pointless.

A lot of people didn't know for months that I was doing breast cancer treatment; this speaks to how self-absorbed many of them were, how little my appearance changed in the early months, or how uninterested they were in gossiping about me. Whatever.

One of the producers who did know about my situation thoughtfully offered to get me "therapeutic grade" pot to take the edge off my nausea during chemo. I passed, somewhat reluctantly. It was very tempting, but it seemed wrong on so many levels.

Hey, at least he made a specific offer of help.

Help Us Help You

As eager as I was to put the breast cancer experience behind me, and not let it define me for the rest of my life, I do want to stay connected with other women who are going through it and help in any way I can. Actually, Courtney put it very well on her blog, while discussing why she remains active in the breast cancer support community, instead of moving on, as so many people expected her to do when her treatment was over.

*A friend . . . described finishing treatment for cancer as
like coming back from a long, horrible trip and getting
off the plane. You walk out only to find your friends and
family have already left the airport. Just when you're
done, and you need support almost more than you ever
did, many in your life will assume it's over. That it's
time to grab some dinner at Chili's and talk about other
things.*

*I consider it my duty—actually, my honor, really—
to be there waiting for people when they get off that
plane.*

So there you have it. You absolutely have to ask for
help, all you type A personalities, Superwomen, and shrink-
ing violets who don't want to be any trouble. If you don't,
you're screwing the rest of us out of a chance to pay back
our debt. And you can't do that to us—we've had cancer, for
chrissakes.

A Lesson Not Learned from Breast Cancer

"I would encourage women to ask for what you need.
Women expect husbands to read their minds. We put aside
our own needs to take care of everybody else and time and
time again our needs are lost, so I would encourage women
to explicitly communicate what you need because you can
get it. You need to tell me how you need to be treated. For

example, if for you knowledge is power, I will show you studies and tell you my reasons, and defend, if necessary, why I chose this path for you. Or maybe I'll say, 'You seem really afraid, and you need a strong competent doctor to take you by the hand. I will be your beacon and you can let go.' Or if you need me to position myself as merely your adviser, then fine, I'll offer my suggestions and I'll defer to you. Whatever you need, you need to tell me."

—Dr. Bonni Gearhart, oncologist

Chapter Six

Sex and the Single (Breasted) Girl

It took nearly a full year for much of the swelling in my breast to go down, and it was probably the only part of me that did during that period, if you catch my drift. Throughout all the months of my treatments, my husband, Dennis, was very supportive and loving. He did seem to avoid contact with the battered breast, which was fine by me. When the breast finally resolved itself into its current shape, I asked him what he thought about it.

"We never really talk about your feelings about my breast," I mentioned to him one day.

"What's the point?" He shrugged. "It is what it is, right?"

And then he asked me whether the flesh that had been removed would ultimately grow back and fill in the divot.

"What am I, a starfish? A newt?" I snapped. "Humans don't grow new body parts when they lose them."

And to think he went to Yale.

We haven't talked about it much since then. . . .

It's so lovely, so romantic, when your husband still finds you desirable and wants to have sex during and right after treatment. But upon deeper consideration, there are two ways of looking at it. Let's face it, you know you look like crap—*you* wouldn't do you—so what does that say about him? That he loves you no matter what you look like, or that he's such an old horn dog that he'll even screw you when your skin is green and your head is bald and he knows perfectly well that sex is the last thing on *your* mind? My husband swears he is a deeply sensitive and enlightened man who found me just as sexy as ever. He even says most of that with a straight face.

I have yet to meet a woman who's gone through treatment who said, "Oh, yeah, the sex was totally incredible. Couldn't do it enough."

If you're out there, please, identify yourself and tell us all your secret.

Sexuality during and even after breast cancer is definitely not just about the breasts. It's more complicated than having to decide whether or not to renovate your bustline. First, of course, is just the way you feel. There's a description some women use for breast cancer treatment, which is "slash, burn, and poison." Your body has been through some if not all three of those, and maybe has the chemical effects of hormone therapy to take into account as well. You're sore, you're exhausted, and you're not necessarily thinking, *You know, what I could really go for is a good old-fashioned roll in the hay.*

Who would want to have sex under those circumstances?

Oh, right. Your partner does.

Duty Booty

It's hard not to think of it sometimes as duty booty, though. If your partner is being affectionate and tender, and finds you desirable, you don't want to tell him that, and this is nothing personal, you'd rather eat raw pork than have sex on that particular occasion. With anybody.

According to some of the cancer experts, you're "supposed to" opt for hugging, kissing, back rubs, and other kinds of physical affection that aren't, strictly speaking, S-E-X, but it never occurred to me to ask if we could take the Chinese menu approach and do some substitutions. It was all or nothing for us, and more "nothing" than "all" during chemotherapy.

Long after your treatment is over, your libido may still be low or nonexistent. There are some drugs and creams that may help. But in my highly unscientific survey, those of us who get sticky and sweaty from hot flashes are not often desperate to get sticky and sweaty from sex. Some hot flashes are caused by hormone therapy like tamoxifen, in a condition also known as chemopause. And if you take a drug like tamoxifen, you may find your sexual appetite has become an anorexic. On the other hand, if you *are* in the mood for sex, and your vagina didn't get the memo, you can have a major issue with dryness.

Now we all want to feel younger, especially during sex, but reliving the first time you had it—"Is it in? Why won't it go in? I don't know, maybe there's something wrong"—is not exactly a recipe for ecstasy. And if you've had radiation, I can tell you from personal experience that your breast does not want to be squashed down by a heavy, sweaty chest pressed against it.

Nothing says good lovin' like a high-pitched, "Yeeoow. Get off my boob," shrieked directly into your partner's ear.

Love me tender, or else.

It might be better to have a conversation about it before it comes to that.

I know what you're thinking: *You mean I really have to tell my partner not to put too much pressure on that area?*

Is your partner a guy?

If so, then I'm thinking the answer is, "Sadly, yes." Not at first, of course, but after it starts to look like it's healed, he might forget how sensitive it still is in the heat of the moment.

It always surprises me that people who can talk about somebody else's sex life night and day so often clam up when it comes to telling their partners what they really want and need. Look at it this way: If you don't talk about how you're feeling, your partner can't possibly know what you need. He'll get it wrong and you'll end up resenting him, even though you know it's not fair.

When men have sexual performance issues because of surgery for prostate cancer, they take Viagra. It will shock you to learn that there is no little blue pill for women's libido problems after breast cancer. For a while, it was thought that testosterone cream applied to the vagina would help, but a Mayo Clinic study in 2007 disproved that. The report I read recommended that doctors do a full evaluation of their patients, and look for vaginal dryness, depression, early menopause, and hormonal imbalance.

Really, Doc? Why do you think she came to see you?

Without getting too far into my bedroom, I will say that for the most part, I've adjusted to the side effects of tamoxifen, including the ones related to sex. It took a long time, but eventually we got back to normal.

The Naked and the Dread

As annoying as it is to try to deal with a sex drive that's stuck in Park, imagine the challenge for young single women who have their libidos and want to get back into the dating pool. How and when do you broach the subject of your breast cancer adventure with a potential new partner?

It would be great if there were an Internet dating site

for post–breast cancer patients, a place where you can adver-
tise what ya want, what ya got, and also what you're missing,
so there are no unpleasant surprises. Or Craigslist: "Single-
breasted woman seeks lover with double vision for conversation, love and laughs." For the reconstructed woman: "Brand
New Breasts need taking out for test drive. Care to go for a
spin?"

On Craigslist, those ads wouldn't even stand out as unusual.

The television writer Courtney Bugler is a young, married woman, so the dating game is not one she has to concern herself with. But after her lumpectomy and treatments,
she struggled with sexuality and self-esteem. It wasn't
about the breast—it was about almost everything else.

"I'm not one of those people who thinks that her breasts
are the key to her sexuality. I had a healthy attitude about
my body. I was a little chubbier than I wanted to be, but I
looked okay.

"But cancer has changed my body. I look at myself and
it isn't me. The 'me' is a size six with long blonde hair, not
size twelve with crazy chemo curls. It's a real adjustment to
look in the mirror and say, this is me, at least for now.

"The challenge is getting your mojo back. How do you
get to feeling good about your body again? That's my biggest issue."

She said she never expected that getting her self-esteem

back would be the hardest part of dealing with the aftermath of breast cancer, but it really stole her self-confidence.

So Courtney did what any of us might do. She started taking pole dancing classes.

"The very first class I went to, we were all supposed to walk and run our fingers through our hair. I was bald. I was just walking in a circle and it hit me how uncomfortable I was in my own skin. I would always feel sexy before, in a situation like that, but I had all these doubts that I couldn't get rid of. I couldn't stop focusing on the bad parts. Finally, as I was driving home, I thought, *Wow, cancer has really fucked me up.* And that pissed me off—that I sort of allowed that to happen."

If I'd had that conversation with myself in the car, I'm pretty sure my next stop would have involved a drive-thru window and a large order of onion rings. But Courtney is clearly a better woman than I. For one thing, she went back to class.

"I love my class," she told me. "There are girls of all sizes in it, and they know what I've been through, and they're very supportive and they've definitely made me feel more comfortable. My husband gave me a stripper pole for my thirtieth birthday and I can go upside down on it."

Wow. I never had that much mojo in my life. You couldn't get me to do a pole dance if I was alone and drunk. But I think it's fantastic that Courtney is bringing sexy back, as Justin Timberlake would put it, by walking the walk and strutting the strut.

Courtney, and pole dancers everywhere, know they deserve to be loved and admired, and maybe even to have a twenty stuffed into their panties. What's sexier than that, I ask you?

The Bald and the Beautiful

We are almost as obsessed with our hair as we are with our breasts in this country—ask any guy who's bald. At least since the 1950s, when greasers gummed their hair back with proto-metrosexual hair product, and the Beatles-inspired hair revolution of the '60s, we've defined ourselves to some extent by our hair. Baby boomers grew up with commercial slogans like, "If I have only one life to live, let me live it as a Blonde," and "Blondes Have More Fun," and "Which Twin Had the Toni?" (which was a home perm commercial but sounds like secret Breast Cancer Club code for asking about a mastectomy).

Think about the huge brouhaha in the media when Britney Spears shaved her head. It was practically considered self-mutilation. And yet nobody said too much about it when, judging by her panty-free crotch flashes earlier in that particular shame spiral, she showed she'd already done the same thing to her vajayjay and was just working her way up.

And lest we forget, for centuries, one of the surest ways

to publicly humiliate a woman was to hack off her hair. You've seen pictures of French women shaved bald by angry mobs because they were Nazi collaborators. Those French really knew how to chop away at a girl's self-esteem. I had the same experience with a French hair stylist at a snooty Manhattan salon once.

One of my first rebellions against joining Cancer Club came when I had to contemplate losing all my hair. As I considered whether to do what everybody else did—just get in line to take the AC/T therapy that would make all my hair fall out—or go with the other, endless chemo that merely thinned my hair, I really felt the pressure to shut up and take my medicine, literally. More than a few people implied that I was being silly to worry about being temporarily bald. And yet, it wasn't silly to me at all.

You know how beautiful Sinéad O'Connor looks as a bald woman in the video where she's singing "Nothing Compares 2 U"?

That wouldn't be me.

I wouldn't be one of the women who looks so beautiful when she's completely bald that you wonder for a moment if she's making a fashion statement. I wanted to go to work, see my friends, attend school functions with my daughter, and concentrate on anything and everything except breast cancer. But I knew I couldn't do that if I was rockin' a wig, and penciling in eyebrows.

When I chose the chemo that spared much of my hair,

every day was a bad hair day, but at least it was *my* bad hair. And it faked out virtually everybody. The response I got most from surprised people when they finally learned what was up with me was, "But you've got hair!" The fact that my skin was greenish, I had lost a lot of weight rapidly, and that the hair I had hung in thin, lifeless strands was completely overlooked. It just goes to show you how important your hair is to the overall impression you're making in the world.

I wonder what it said to the world when I showed up for the first day of kindergarten sporting those awful, mid-forehead Mamie Eisenhower bangs? I shudder to think.

During chemo I developed an almost OCD-like penchant for constantly running my fingers through my hair and counting the number of strands that came out each time. After a few months I had a bald spot in the back; luckily I couldn't see it, although my husband and daughter helpfully informed me when it appeared. Dr. Chuang told me recently she was surprised by how much hair I lost, but kind of relieved.

"We like to see some evidence that the patient really is taking all her pills," she said and chuckled.

I had great blood counts almost the entire time I was on chemo, and more than once I thought I noticed her eyeing me a little suspiciously.

The producer Fiona Conway dreaded losing her hair to chemo so much that she inadvertently caused herself what I can only describe as a case of premature baldness.

"When I was first diagnosed—about the second thing into my head was 'Oh my God, I'm going to be bald,' " she told me.

"What happens, though, is that from the time of diagnosis until you lose your hair is about four to six weeks. So I really had time to prepare. I convinced myself that hair wasn't so important. I got a divorce from my hair."

But only a few days into the chemotherapy she began to look for signs of hair loss.

"As soon as my hair started to shed—about two weeks after the first chemo—I jumped the gun and had my head buzzed. I ended up having a healthy amount of buzz-cut hair for another three weeks."

Fiona couldn't bring herself to spend a lot of money on a good human hair wig, which can cost several thousand dollars. For most women, it's just not an affordable option.

"I decided that I would rather spend thousands on a great trip or a piece of art or jewelry than on something I was going to not wear again, I hope, after a few months, and something that symbolized a painful episode in my life," she told me.

"I opted for a synthetic. I had it cut, styled, and fitted. But I have hated this wig from day one. It's hot, it feels like I'm wearing a swim cap, and it's itchy, and the hair is icky to the touch. I felt from the first moment I wore it in public that it screamed, 'Wig—person in a wig!' Anyone I had eye contact with on the train or subway, I assumed, was wondering why the hell I was wearing that ugly wig!"

I saw her in that wig, by the way, and I don't remember having to stifle the impulse to scream, "Wig!" I understand that it was awful to wear, but it wasn't nearly as obvious as it felt to her. In any case, she was eventually able to ditch the fake wig for a real one.

"I inherited a human hair wig from a very kind woman who didn't need it anymore. When I put it on, it immediately changed my life! I know that sounds dramatic, but it really did. I took it to my stylist, who said to me, 'I'll make you look like yourself,' and he did. I walked out of his salon on top of the world. No blaring 'wig' announcements!

"I feel like me again. It's comfortable, it moves, I can even feel the wind in my hair. Lesson learned . . . spend the money if you can," Fiona advises.

Or hope that a rich friend needs chemo.

The Question Inquiring Minds Want to Know but Are Afraid to Ask

When I lost more than half my hair over the months of chemo, I still had enough to get by, although my flat, stringy hair hung as lifelessly as a cheap wig. My normally long eyelashes got stubbier, but extra mascara took care of that. On the other hand, my legs and armpits were as smooth as a baby's tushie. No hair, no stubble, no shaving. And I had the bikini line of a porn star. I was more than a little disappointed when it eventually grew back.

That's what you wanted to know, right? Among the Frequently Asked Questions of chemo patients, I've learned, is, "Um, do you mind if I ask, do you lose all your hair . . . on your whole body?"

Most of us are too polite, or too taken aback, to reply, "Do you mean is my hoo-hoo as hairless as a naked mole rat?"

Not that you deserve to know if you're not going through it yourself, but in the interest of science and public service, I will tell you.

The answer is, "Yeah, pretty much."

On the chemo I was doing, and from what I've learned comparing notes with others, it's a gradual process. Your vagina reappears from its years in hiding through what we call "a slow reveal" in television terms.

Kind of like Geraldo's prime-time special in which he opened Al Capone's (empty) vault. And given the sad state of my libido at the time, about as big a letdown.

A Lesson Not Learned from Breast Cancer

"My appearance has always been on my mind. I always want to look my best, and that didn't change when I was undergoing chemo, although I didn't really look like myself. Steroids puffed out my face, and without hair on my head, eyebrows and lashes, I looked rather scary. For a time I avoided all the mirrors in my home. Even so, whenever I went to chemo I always put on a little extra bronzer and blush. It was the only thing I could control. I wanted to look better than I felt."

—Gloria, attorney, real estate broker

Chapter Seven

When the Patient Isn't

> ## Lesson Five:
>
> Patience is a highly overrated
> virtue; if you demand instant
> results you may not get
> them instantly, but you'll get
> them faster than you would
> have by waiting patiently.

The First Radiation Patient

In 1896, just months after the discovery of X-rays, Mrs. Rose Lee of Philadelphia, who had an inoperable tumor in her left breast, became the first person to receive radiation treatment for breast cancer. Treatment involved putting an X-ray tube directly against the lesion. While her tumor shrank following two and a half weeks of radiation exposure, the treatment did not save her. She died months later. Still, doctors impatient to find a way to use X-rays to kill cancer cells persevered, sometimes at the cost of their own lives. Many of the researchers experimenting with X-rays to find the proper dose died of leukemia themselves.

X-ray Visions

The doctor who had tried to treat Rose Lee probably knew her chances of being cured by radiation weren't good, but he had run out of other ideas, and had nothing to lose.

I can relate. I often do my clearest thinking at my wit's end. Exasperation turns to inspiration; it forces me to find a different way to think about a problem, and sometimes to choose an alternate route to reach my goal.

By the time I got to radiation, my goal was simple. I had been dealing with cancer treatment for more than seven months and I had had enough. I knew going in to the whole treatment process that it was going to be a challenge for me to stay with it. I can be very patient when it comes to waiting for a good thing to happen, but I'm not so good at enduring unpleasant situations like, say, cancer. Or radiation; five days a week for seven weeks was not my idea of fun—and getting there meant braving a long walk from the subway to the hospital during a brutally cold February and early March. More than once I wished I had been able to have that one-week mammosite radiation therapy that I had planned on before surgery.

Now, before you can even begin radiation, there is a lot of pre-treatment work to be done. Technicians and doctors have to map out exactly where to aim their rays. This is the simulation phase, and it includes such sophisticated high-tech techniques as taking a felt-tip pen and marking up your breast into sections that look like "choice cuts" until you resemble a steer on a butcher shop chart. When they get you positioned exactly right, they make a kind of body mold that you will lie on to ensure that you're precisely where you're supposed to be on the death ray table. And then they tattoo you with little spots. No kidding. They really do that, as a guide.

I thought the doctor was joking at first when she told me they'd be tattooing me; it seemed so primitive, especially in a state-of-the-art facility. *Gosh, why not just make a voodoo doll in my image and put that thing on the radiation table?* I thought.

And then I got annoyed. I didn't relish the whole concept of having six or eight dark spots tattooed on my already not-so-great-looking chest, and I had had more than enough of needles. So I rebelled. I questioned authority. I asked, politely, if this was really necessary.

My surprised radiation oncologist chuckled, but she told me I was free to negotiate a better deal with the technicians if I could, and then she left the room. And it turned out the technicians decided they could get it right with two tattoo spots, instead of six or eight. That's what I got. Over the long weeks that followed, I never found anybody else who raged against the tattoo machine, but I did find plenty of women who wished it had occurred to them, too.

Until I met Jacqueline Skaggs, that is. She refused to get tattooed at all, so she beats me. For both of us, it was a matter of empowerment.

"It felt like my first chance to grab back control over my body," she says. "It might seem silly, but it was great to say no to the doctors."

Sometimes the technicians teased me for making their work more complicated, and sometimes I did feel a bit guilty, just for a minute. But I was impatient to capture back a little shred of dignity in an otherwise most undignified situation.

Actually, my impatience got me more than my dignity. It got me into radiation weeks ahead of schedule. The usual protocol requires a patient to finish chemo and rest a bit before starting radiation, but since my blood counts were normal until nearly the very end of chemo, I began to think I could handle both simultaneously. I did some research and found that occasionally it's done. To my delight, Dr. Chuang said yes to letting me double up on treatments. I only saved myself a few weeks, but at that point, just believing I was gaming the system was enough to lift my spirits. I would have done anything to finish early.

On the Road Back to Healthyville

Radiation is like the cease-fire that precedes a peace treaty in a war; during the cease-fire nobody's trying to kill you anymore but you can't go back home to your normal life yet. Still, the fact that there are no longer bullets whizzing past you means you can lift your head up out of the trenches and take a moment to consider where you are in the landscape of your inner self.

And what I found, to my profound relief, was that I felt very much like the same person I had been when all the trouble started. I thought for sure I was heading straight back to my old place in Healthyville, only slightly worse for wear. And as I traveled, I picked up little neurotic parts of myself that I'd left by the wayside when they became too exhausting to carry while I was coping with breast cancer. One of the first I came across was that little part of me that likes to check out the competition to see if I'm missing anything.

Having a competitive streak is good if you're fighting for television ratings, or real estate, or the last piece of pie. But I'm not sure how it fits in to breast cancer recovery. Yet, for some slightly embarrassing reason, I became aware of the need to be doing breast cancer the best. After months of keeping to myself, I was kibitzing with every patient I encountered, and while I think I just seemed chatty, I was actually checking them out. I compared my progress with theirs—jealous of the ones who were much further along than I was, glad that I was better off than some others, quizzing everybody about their doctors and their treatment and how they were feeling. I needed to believe that I was doing everything the best possible way. I didn't want to flunk breast cancer treatment.

Why? Why was this so important to me? Hard to say, but I do know that it felt good to try to excel at something, anything, after all those months of just barely getting through. Besides, radiation was so boring I had to make a game of it to motivate myself to finish.

I also wanted to make certain I wasn't missing out on any opportunity to improve my situation. For example, if I'd met Jacqueline Skaggs and learned that she had managed to get away without doing any tattoo dots at all, I would have been really upset with myself. Luckily by the time I did meet her, I was over it.

It could be that when the dust, and my stomach, settled, I was just the same old bat-shit crazy person I'd always been. But it's not as though I was the only one playing a round of Survivor: Breast Cancerland. This was all happening in New York, after all, and mostly on the Upper East Side, the breeding ground of assertive uber-bitch Ladies Who Lunch (on Each Other's Livers). I ran into a radiation waiting room buddy by the coat rack one cold Monday morning and was filled with envy and grudging admiration as she regaled me with the story of her exhilarating return to the slopes. She'd spent the whole weekend skiing in Vermont.

Skiing? Are you kidding?

I considered it a physical triumph to walk six blocks to the subway and six blocks back every morning.

Did I recover from my jealousy by mentioning how glad I was that she'd gone when she did because when she was at *my* stage of radiation—just a few more to go, hah!—she'd probably be too tired?

Or did I just think about saying it, and instead graciously express my admiration for her athleticism and stamina? Hmmm ... can't be sure.

Looking back on it, this was an obvious sign that breast cancer was not going to result in a personality makeover for me, even if I could use one.

Not that I wasn't generally very supportive of the other women on Radiation Row, especially the ones who were also rushing off to work after getting zapped. I enjoyed chatting in the waiting room with the other women coming to the end of their breast cancer forced march. We were champing at the bit to get the hell out of there, talked about our work and our kids, and groaned about the long waits to see the doctor for our weekly checkups. As our health returned we grew ever more impatient to get back to our lives. I wished I could be the first one back, with the fewest changes in my life. Chemo felt like I had cancer; radiation just felt like I was stuck in a traffic jam.

I didn't take it seriously. And I forgot for a while that some other women did. Some get really scared.

While having a cancer chat one day with an architect in the waiting area, I noticed a young woman across from us shifting uncomfortably in her chair. I asked her if she was all right. She wasn't. Our conversation was making her extremely anxious. We were her equivalent of a live chat room she didn't want to be in—actually, we were literally a chat room—and it was giving her an anxiety attack. She obviously was trying to be patient and wait us out, but she was suffering for it. We felt awful and changed the subject immediately, of course. I only wish I'd noticed her distress sooner, or that she'd just told us to zip it. I wish she hadn't been so damned polite and, well, patient.

She had discovered a lump a few months after having a baby. I didn't know if she was nursing the baby, and it would have been wrong to ask, but it made me think about my own pregnancy and the way I felt about my breasts at that time.

My attitude changed when mine ceased to be purely decorative sex toys and became, temporarily, the source of nourishment for my tiny infant. My breasts went from being costars to leading ladies, divas who demanded and got tons of attention. In the first days after Julia was born, my breasts ruled my entire life. I was always either nursing, pumping, or worrying about leakage. (There must be twenty pictures of me as a bleary-eyed new mother, smiling at the camera while oblivious to the telltale wet spots spreading across my blouse.) My breasts were a lot more powerful than I'd ever known, and they deserved, and got, my respect.

I can only imagine how I would have felt back then if I'd learned that a tumor was lurking in one of them.

When you undergo radiation therapy, you have to lie down on the table, open your gown, and bare your wounded breast while technicians in another room manipulate a moving radiation machine. The technicians are nice; they make small talk as they carefully adjust your body on the table, move your gown farther away from your breast, place your arm where it won't be in the way. But the experience itself, in which you are lying there, alone, breast exposed, is dehumanizing, no matter how much the staff tries to connect with you.

If you've recently regarded that vulnerable breast as the source for nurturing a new baby, it must be awful to have to expose it to radiation. (Fortunately, it's very rare to get breast cancer while nursing. Lumps are common, and scary, but usually caused by blocked milk ducts. Still, they need to be checked out.)

It's interesting that during treatment, this young woman was my only reminder of the whole reason we have breasts in the first place.

What I learned about radiation:

First and foremost, for most women, it's a piece of cake compared to chemo—no nausea, no feeling crappy.

Some women who are still recovering from the whacking their bodies endured during chemo definitely feel fatigued. I didn't.

It just takes a few minutes but it's quite boring.

Your breast and surrounding area can get "sunburned" after a few weeks. There are some superstrength moisturizing creams that help with that. Some women get really crispy, but I was lucky just to have a moderate sunburn-like effect.

Your doctor might tell you to lay off the antioxidants, because they may interfere with the radiation. So if you normally pound Pom (the pomegranate juice) cocktails or eat gigantic amounts of broccoli, you have to change your habits temporarily.

Oh, and by the way: Your breast may be tender for a long time. As in, forever. In my unscientific survey of dozens of women, nobody was warned that years later their boobs would still hurt, and *everybody's* boobs still hurt. It's not that big a deal, but radiation does seem to be the gift that keeps on giving. Especially when it's time to get a mammogram again, and my always tender breast gets twisted counterclockwise (or maybe it's clockwise, but what the hell difference does it make—it hurts) before being squished flat in a vise so the doctors can see around the scar tissue from my surgery. I grit my teeth and bear it, though, because at least I still have that breast.

The Impatient Patient

I know so many women who say, "Breast cancer taught me to slow down, stop and smell the roses, enjoy the moment." Really?

If anything, it taught me that there's not a moment to waste. I was even impatient in the chemo room, despite how much I dreaded the needle. If I had to wait a long time to get hooked up to the poison machine, I did a lot of subtle things, like looking at my watch and sighing. I think I even muttered, "Tick, tock, ladies," under my breath once. They were a great group of caring professionals who did their utmost to make us all as comfortable as they could. In my case, that meant getting me in and out as fast as humanly possible.

Impatience really is my burden and my blessing. The good thing about it is it creates a mind-set where I try to anticipate what will slow me down before it happens, and often I'm able to develop a plan that allows me to avoid roadblocks. The bad thing is that when I can't avoid roadblocks and I do get slowed down, I can be a little irrational. What can I say? I'm working on it. I try to tell myself to relax, breathe, remember that nothing terrible will happen if I am delayed for a few minutes. But I can't honestly say that breast cancer, or any other experience I've had, has helped me make much progress in the pursuit of "serenity now."

Three years after cancer, I will still walk in and then immediately out of three or four consecutive Starbucks if there are long lines, no matter how much I want coffee. Luckily, there's a zoning regulation in New York that requires a Starbucks on every other corner in Manhattan.

Why Can't We Go from Nun's Disease to None's Disease?

More than anything, though, I am extremely impatient with the lack of progress being made on breast cancer prevention.

From the fourteenth century to not so very long ago, breast cancer was called the Nun's Disease, because nuns got it at a far higher rate than the female population at large. Unfortunately, over the last forty years American women have caught up with our Sisters. Now, about 12 percent of us will have breast cancer at some point in our lives. So, I guess we can eliminate "becoming a nun" from the list of potential causes of breast cancer. But that's not much progress, is it?

If it's no longer the Nun's Disease, what is it? Some would call it the Feminist Disease. Whether or not you blame feminism, and the emphasis on higher education and careers over staying home and having babies, the fact is, women today do have fewer babies, have them later in life, and breast-feed them for shorter periods of time than our grandmothers did. That exposes our bodies to more estrogen, and estrogen fuels many breast cancer tumors. If further proof of the connection between estrogen exposure and breast cancer were needed, it was provided in 2006, when a sharp drop in breast cancer rates was attributed to the large number of women getting off the hormone replacement therapy they'd been taking. (And, of course, they got off HRT because, despite what doctors had previously told them, it didn't protect them from heart disease and it did expose them to higher cancer risks.)

The good news is that early detection and better treatments are allowing more women to beat the disease. Of all the millions of cancer survivors in the United States, breast cancer survivors are by far the largest group, and the treatments get better every year. The bad news, though, is that nobody knows precisely why so many more women get breast cancer today than one generation ago.

And while there has been enormous progress in the treatment of the disease, much of the good news applies only to older women, as Courtney Bugler pointed out to me.

"Everybody talks about twenty-year survival rates and statistics for twenty years. But I'm not just trying to have a good life for twenty or thirty years. Twenty years would only get me to forty-eight. Sometimes when I hear those statistics I clench up and say to myself, 'Yeah, but you're not trying to beat this for fifty or sixty years. *I* am.' In fact, I think I have to operate under the assumption that I *will* get cancer again. It doesn't freak me out, but if I live to be eighty or ninety years old, well, fifty years is a lot of time to live without ever getting cancer again. It could happen."

This is what's so frustrating. For all the breakthroughs in treatment, we're not much better at understanding the prevention or causes of breast cancer than when it was the Nun's Disease.

As if that weren't maddening enough, public health policy is confusing and contradictory. When is the appropriate age to begin mammogram screening? Depends on whom you listen to, and what they are taking into consideration. Should women do breast self-examination every month, as we've been told for years, or are they of no real help in reducing deaths? Should tamoxifen be used prophylactically by women at higher risk of developing breast cancer, despite known potential side effects like blood clots and uterine cancer?

For forty thousand women every year in the United States alone, there comes a point when the words on that first known medical journal, written in about 1500 BC, are still true today: "There is no treatment."

So can you blame me for being impatient? Especially when you go over the list of what we actually do know for sure about preventing breast cancer.

After all, there *are* some known risk factors. Being a woman is the biggest risk factor. Getting old is almost as dangerous; the older you are, the more likely you'll get it. If you have close female relatives who have had breast cancer, your risk increases, although about 90 percent of us have no family history of it. If you don't have babies, or you have them relatively late in life, and if you don't breast-feed them, you increase your risk. If you're overweight, if you eat red meat, if you drink too much alcohol, you increase your risk. If you eat processed meats, you're at greater risk for cancer. (Actually, I always thought those pimento loaf sandwiches my mother fed us as kids were lethal, but that's another story.)

So, here's what I can infer that the medical profession would recommend if you want to have the best chance of avoiding breast cancer. Don't be born a woman. If you are, have a lot of babies, breast-feed them 'til they're old enough to drive, don't have a mother or sister who had it, and don't get old. Oh, and stay away from bars and barbecues.

There, that's simple, isn't it?

Now you see why I'm impatient, despite all the positive statistics about survival.

Impatience was a core trait of my character before I got breast cancer and it's a core trait to this day. And that's part of the one big lesson I did learn from breast cancer.

A Lesson Not Learned from Breast Cancer

"What got me through breast cancer, twice, was trusting my own beliefs and ideologies about how to define my femininity and womanliness vis-à-vis mastectomy in a breast-obsessed world. I got this persistence and stubbornness from my mother, not from breast cancer. I trust my intuition and common sense. You've got nothing to lose by going with your gut. And don't buy into the idea that you have to have a positive disposition all the time. You have to have the freedom to bitch."

—Jacqueline Skaggs, artist, designer

Part Three

THE AFTER
(CANCER)
LIFE

Chapter Eight

The One Big Lesson I Learned

Lesson Six:

Breast cancer doesn't change
who you are, it confirms
who you are.

When I discovered that I had breast cancer, I had just begun a project that I considered to be both mission-based (launching a radio network to try to effect a political change) and, potentially, a lot of fun. You don't have to agree with my politics to understand that I treasured the opportunity to do work that I believed mattered. In some ways it was a huge risk, walking away from thirty years in the traditional news business to launch a new media company, especially since I am and have always been the primary financial support of our family. But change had always been an important part of my career; I get bored quickly and need new challenges. As it turned out, I was surrounded by the smartest and funniest people I'd ever worked with, we did have an impact on the political dialogue in the nation, and my two years at Air America were undoubtedly the most fun I'd ever had at work.

Two years after completing breast cancer treatment, I was at it again, launching a new company with a former television colleague. This time it's a Web site that has nothing to do with politics but does take advantage of my many years producing informational programming. Again I'm risking financial security, working long hours, and insisting on having fun.

Throughout it all, I have been able to count on the love and support of my family, who are great at jumping in when needed to get us out of any mess I get us into. My daughter is working at least two jobs while in college, and my husband has a way of working wonders with diminishing amounts of money; I trade in our milk cow for three magic beans, and he sighs and then climbs the resulting beanstalk to see if he can't find a goose that lays golden eggs. So far, no goose, but at least nobody's been eaten by a giant ogre shouting "fee fi fo fum."

The point is, no matter what happens, we try to keep on keeping on, making adjustments that still fit the pattern of our lives. We like our lives. While I was traveling through the dark and creepy tunnel of breast cancer treatment, I did what most women with breast cancer do—I tried to maintain the normal routines of our lives as much as possible. When a friend called to tell me that she'd asked Julia how I was, and Julia replied, "She's just my mom . . . crazy as ever," I was thrilled.

Meanwhile, the world outside was going on as it always had. It was fast, it was stressful, it was challenging, and it was exhausting. And when I was finally able to rejoin it, it was a relief.

I was thrilled to be able to go back to the same issues I've been dealing with for my whole life. Unlike many ex—cancer patients, including some I've interviewed in this book, I can't say that I no longer let the little problems of life upset me as much, or that I've got a greater perspective on what's really important. I *do* sweat the small stuff, still. The small stuff adds up to the big picture that is my life. I don't think what mattered to me before cancer was frivolous or foolish, and if anything, a close encounter with cancer makes me care twice as much about the big and small "stuff." I may be in a new, slightly altered package, but I'm concentrated now, and unwilling to waste a drop of my time. This, too, is the same attitude I had before—it's breast cancer, once again, confirming who I am, not changing me.

Which is not to say that breast cancer had no impact on my life. In some ways it was like a slap in the face, the kind that in B movies resulted in the slapped person saying, "Thanks. I needed that."

You won't hear me saying "thanks." I didn't need that, not any of it. I didn't need to be told that life is short (because it really isn't; it's just that our to-do lists are so long and we waste a lot of time); I didn't need to be reminded to tell my family I love them every time we say good-bye (we did that before and we do it still); and I damn sure didn't need to be made aware of how unprepared I was to see myself as a middle-aged person. Having breast cancer forced me to admit that I'd been deluding myself into thinking that I was still young and had endless options. And even though I never believed that breast cancer would kill me, I was keenly aware that having a serious health issue is one of those things that usually happens when you get . . . um, older.

God, how I hate that. I still want to believe that my future is like a completely clear blue sky, with "unlimited visibility," as the pilots say. It makes me sad, and angry, to be forced to acknowledge that some windows of opportunity have closed (I guess it's time to cross "lead singer of a girl band" off my Life List) and that I ~~may be~~ am middle-aged. I wasn't ready for middle age, but breast cancer pulled me into it, kicking and screaming.

Was this the takeaway message for me, that I should acknowledge my age, and plan accordingly?

Screw that.

The Big Lesson I learned from breast cancer was something else entirely, something that seems so obvious now, but it took me a long time to come to it.

The Epiphany of No Epiphany

One night, when a year had passed since the completion of my treatment and the meaning of life still had not revealed itself to me, I ran into a friend, the artist Jill Levine, at a party. She had had a mastectomy more than a year before my cancer, and seemed to have escaped psychologically unscathed. In fact, her life appeared to be exactly as it was before cancer. I wanted to know whether she felt the same way I did, and if so, did she feel like something was lacking?

"I gotta tell you, Jill," I admitted, "I don't feel any different now than I did before I had breast cancer. I've waited for more than a year, and . . . nothing. I don't know what's wrong with me, but I don't think it changed me at all."

She just chuckled.

"Nothing's wrong with you," she said. "It didn't change me, either. I had cancer, they removed it, and that was it. I was done. Same thing for you. Why should it change you? Stop looking for something that isn't there."

I was pretty surprised. I'd never heard anybody say that before.

"So that's it? You had cancer, and then you didn't? Just like that?" I asked.

She seemed so calm, so matter-of-fact about it.

"Well, I was totally freaked out when the doctor first recommended a mastectomy," she said. "I just couldn't believe I needed surgery. But then I thought, *Okay, I can make myself crazy or I can just accept the fact that I have it and they'll fix it and then that will be that.* Life goes on."

Just like that. So here it was, the big discovery. I always thought you had to climb a mountain in Tibet and visit a reclusive wise man to learn the Meaning of Life. But maybe the meaning of breast cancer can be found while drinking wine and leaning against a wall in a SoHo loft. The epiphany is that there is no epiphany. Cancer is simply cancer, and it's quite enough to get through it and move on.

Jill was a fundamentally optimistic woman before breast cancer, during treatment, and then after it. It wasn't a transformational experience; it simply clarified for her who and what she was.

To what did she owe this serene attitude about breast cancer? I asked her, months later, on the phone.

"When I was five years old my father got a strep infection, which led to kidney disease. From then on, he was always sick. He dealt with dialysis for years, and a kidney transplant, which led to complications that ultimately killed him. But when he got the diagnosis he just carried on with his life. He was a retired policeman, he had a pension, but he continued to work part-time. And he just never let on about what he was going through. He was very stoic. It was an example for me to see that bad things do happen, but you deal with them, you go forward."

But during our conversation I found that it was more than the example her father provided her about handling illness. It was her outlook, overall, about life. It's just her nature to be happy.

"I get disappointed sometimes, of course, but I'm a very positive person. I never once thought breast cancer was a death sentence. I told myself that millions of people go through this, and I'll be able to do it, too. And it was a breast, which I didn't need. As an artist, it would have been far worse if I'd lost an eye or my hand. It happened in the late summer, and I was excited that I would get to extend my summer vacation by six weeks while I was on medical leave. I was in my studio painting for an extra six weeks."

"So you never worry about cancer anymore?" I asked her.

"I did sometimes in the first year or so, you know, when every headache could be a brain tumor, and if my breast was sore from PMS I did worry. And I always get nervous when I'm having my mammogram on the one breast. You know, I only have one breast that could get cancer now, and I don't believe I will, but if I did, they'd remove it, and I know I would go on. I've done it."

And to top it all off, Jill—artist, New York City public school art teacher, fifty-two-year-old woman, and my Breast Cancer Yoda, had achieved what I had only aspired to—she had twenty-minute breast cancer. Surgery, immediate reconstruction, nothing else. No chemo, no radiation, no tamoxifen even.

While her treatment was completely different than mine, her point of view was exactly the same. And if we both felt that way, it was likely that there were other women out there who did, too.

I told a friend, the ABC News executive Amy Entelis, that a year after breast cancer I couldn't think of any way I'd changed.

"You, too?" she asked conspiratorially. "I thought it was just me."

It wasn't just us. I asked Governor Jodi Rell if having breast cancer had changed her life.

"I can't say there's anything fundamentally different. Of course you realize your blessings, but I think I would have done that anyway. Breast cancer didn't change that. I would say 9/11 changed that more. I made a promise to myself that day that I wouldn't hang up the phone without telling a loved one, 'I love you.' I had already started a change in what I think is important."

I asked the theater director Theresa Flais whether she is a different person now that she's had a long, tough battle with breast cancer.

"I don't think so," she said. "I think the only thing that has changed is that I've learned to let things go more easily, things that have affected me negatively. I used to hold on to anger or hurt, but I've learned that's not important, let it go. There's more to life, like my kids and how I feel when I'm with them, than the negative things. Since I made that decision I sleep better, I relax more."

The part-time accountant and full-time wife and mother Vivian McDevitt, who had a double mastectomy and chemotherapy in 2007, told me she learned things from watching her sister go through breast cancer. Vivian was the calmest, most matter-of-fact person I've ever met, even more casual about it than I was.

"It's a disease. If you had a cold you wouldn't say, why

me? You'd eat chicken soup and get better. Twenty years ago it wasn't like that, we all know that, but I knew I would be cured."

As for whether breast cancer treatment has made Vivian a different person than she was before, well, you can probably guess.

"I feel like I'm radically the same. More me than ever before."

A lawyer and real estate agent, Gloria, who went through surgery, chemo, and radiation just months after her mother completed breast cancer treatment, laughed when I asked her if the experience had changed her much.

"Not a whole lot. The person that I was the day before I was diagnosed was the kind of person who had already learned early on to appreciate my life and all that I have. I've always been optimistic and grateful. I know there are some people who were real assholes before cancer, and then it changed them, but I was a nice person before and I didn't need it to make me be nicer."

The soap opera writer and blogger Courtney Bugler surprised herself as she answered the question, "Has breast cancer changed you?"

"In many ways, my life is just the same. During treatment I would have thought that it would never go back to being the same. But I still procrastinate, shop for shoes when I should be working, let the laundry pile up. Now, there is cancer as one part of my life, but a lot of it is the same. I will say that sometimes I stop and think about my life and tell myself, 'You know what, this is good.' I wouldn't have stopped to think about it before."

Breast cancer was not an extreme spiritual makeover for me. It wasn't an opportunity to become wiser, slower, faster, more generous with my time, more selfish with my time. It wasn't a path from one life course to another.

It didn't happen to me for a Good Reason.

I assume it happened for a series of bad reasons. Or maybe it just happened.

There are women who say that cancer improved their lives somehow. There's even a book called *Why I'm Glad I Had Breast Cancer.* I read it. I wasn't glad.

I've often wondered at the determined and relentless pressure to find something good in something so god-awful as breast cancer. No other cancer, including the other women's cancers, carries with it such a loaded set of expectations.

I think sometimes the pressure to live our cancer experience, and its aftermath, on the bright side, is partially self-created. Look how difficult it is for so many of us to ask for help during treatment, because we don't want to be a burden, or to be seen as whiners or weaklings. We want our homes to seem just the same as always; we want to be available to our kids, so they don't worry about us. We want to do for our husbands as much as possible—within limits—and we don't want to inconvenience our friends or the people we work with.

We put on our own happy faces.

I used to joke that it was easier on my life for me to be the one with cancer than if it were Dennis, but I was only half kidding.

Maybe some of us also sense that the pink ribbons have strings attached. No, I'm not saying they really do—but it feels as though there is a subtle social contract between the healthy helpers and the women on whom they're bestowing so much time and money and support that says, "Hey, show up and be a good example for the rest of us. Be positive and brave and upbeat. Give us hope." Even if you reject that notion, just from the perspective of *manners*, for God's sake, if people are going out of their way to walk, and race, and write checks and buy pink stuff for the cause, isn't there some obligation to be grateful and cheerful? To make everybody around you feel better, like all their efforts are worthwhile?

I suspect the determined cheerfulness is just another form of denial, a way of telling yourself, "It's not that bad."

For Me? You Shouldn't Have. No, Really.

Did you ever hear someone, usually a celebrity with access to, well, everything she could ever want or need, describe breast cancer as a gift? The first time I heard it I must confess I was a bit shocked. I had no idea. I'd feel embarrassed—where are my manners—except that I just don't know who I should be thanking for it. (Environmental polluters? My mom and dad? I'm so confused.)

To tell you the truth, when my gift arrived, it seemed more like some junk mail that just sat there waiting for me to pay attention to it, like a five-pound catalogue from an auto parts chain, or the September issue of *Vogue*. If it was a gift, it was even worse than a holiday basket filled with hickory-smoked cheeses and specialty flavored Slim Jim samples.

Then I got to thinking, well, maybe there's a cancer-is-a-gift registry that I didn't even know about. You know, like for brides or mothers-to-be. You probably register online. Let's do it together—it's a little tricky picking out the gift of cancer for someone else, so for this exercise, we'll just say it's for us.

Let's see, of course you'd have to choose a size—and believe me, girls, less is definitely more, so go for Small. Next, pick out the kind of tumor you'd like, and here you see a lot of choices. Whew, makes my head spin. When you're all set with your tumor, you get to choose a nice gift of surgery, something that fits your lifestyle. Now, do you want to be given the gift of chemo? Then don't forget to check that box (it shows you're truly committed!). And if you want radiation, that's a big one, but maybe your friends and family will buy you sets of five, until you've got the full set of thirty-five. It's just like buying place settings of your china or silver pattern! You'll want to register for some insurance, no doubt, and of course, a very good prescription drug plan. All those medications cost money, girls! Thank God for the registry.

I wonder if you can register for those darling yellow warning signs for your car: "Tumor on board."

I never believed the old adage "It's better to give than receive" until I heard about the Gift of Cancer. I mean, we've all gotten crappy gifts from time to time, but if you think cancer is a gift, you must really have a closet full of shitty stuff.

If you think cancer is a gift, I hope you've saved the receipt.

If you truly believe cancer is a gift, you can't come to my next birthday party.

I guess you've figured out that, of all the maddening ways in which people try to search for meaning in the random meaninglessness that is breast cancer, nothing annoys me more than the women who declare that breast cancer is a gift. It's the social pressure to be the Good, Cheerful Survivor, taken to its extreme.

Can't we all get through a life crisis without receiving a gift at the end, to make it "worth" it?

Is diabetes a gift, or heart disease? Or is there only a consolation prize for playing "Who Wants to Be a Breast Cancer Survivor?"

I've said that every woman should do whatever it takes to get herself through breast cancer—it's not up to me or anybody else to judge them.

So, I'm not judging the women who say they're thankful

that they had it, but I am compelled to point out that those women were given the greatest gift of all—good luck. They were lucky enough to have curable cancer. Maybe they consider breast cancer to be a journey of self-awareness or enlightenment, but for tens of thousands of other women every year, it's a journey to tragedy. They're the ones who suffered through multiple rounds of surgeries and chemo, who fought as hard, who were just as brave, who deserved to live just as much, but didn't. Breast cancer was not a gift to them, or to the loved ones they left behind.

I'm certain the heartfelt proclamations about the gift of cancer are meant to be inspirational, and they probably do inspire some women, which is great.

I wonder, though, how many are inspired to believe they *ought* to be inspired, and then try to convince themselves they are. It's a subtle, perhaps unintentional mind game that causes some rational women to doubt or ignore their true feelings. It suggests that if you're not blissed out on breast cancer, well, that's just sad. Poor you.

(Lance Armstrong has called his cancer a gift, but he gets a pass from me, because he does so much good work, political as well as social, to advance the cause of preventing, treating, and curing all kinds of cancers. He doesn't just talk the talk.)

The oncologist Dr. Bonni Gearhart is very optimistic about the future treatment of breast cancer. She believes we're on the brink of huge breakthroughs that will make current treatment seem primitive. But she rejects the happy talk.

"If you really want to call a spade a spade, breast cancer sucks, and there's nothing good about it. I appreciate you want to make lemonade out of lemons, but there is value in truth. And I think it's important to see the good and the bad . . . it's still a gruesome disease."

She's a doctor who sees breast cancer patients every day, so she doesn't have the luxury of ignoring the cold, hard facts.

As for me, I find comfort in knowing the facts, not in faith—I always have, except when the facts are too ugly to contemplate. Then I find comfort in denial. Breast cancer didn't change that about me. It's my basic nature. When I go on a spiritual journey, I tend to get lost.

A Wake-Up Call

When you've finished your treatment, I predict you'll find that breast cancer confirmed who you were, too. You'll know that you're as tough or even tougher than you thought. You'll know you deserve to honor your accomplishment and all the people who helped you achieve it. And you'll come to understand that the challenge that remains is learning how to live with the knowledge that you had breast cancer. It is not uncommon to suffer depression after treatment, and if you even suspect that's the case, ask your oncologist to recommend a therapist who can help you get over it.

Gloria, the forty-six-year-old lawyer and real estate agent who'd had breast cancer just months after her mother completed treatment for it, began to realize she was depressed a few months after her treatment ended.

"Feeling depressed is not part of my nature," she told me, "so to feel sad all the time was overwhelming. I thought, *I'm done with treatment, why am I sad?* But while you're in treatment seeing doctors every week there are people looking after you and checking up and you're so involved with the physical aspects that you don't take the time to think about it. Finally, when you get back to normal, that's when you have time for your brain to process what went on. And that's when it hit me that I went through something painful and disturbing."

Fortunately, she went to a therapist and got help, and now she's fine again.

I know so many women who were depressed after they finished all of their treatments, and not one of them was warned that it might happen, which made them feel even worse until they got help. And the depression doesn't necessarily happen right away. Dr. Mary Jane Massie, a psychiatrist at Memorial Sloan-Kettering, told me that sometimes women virtually "sail through their treatment," psychologically speaking, and don't begin to process what they went through for a year or more after they finish it.

I guess I would qualify as one who sailed through, although I definitely got seasick at times. And when I looked back on the voyage, it was like a Circle Line cruise around Manhattan. I don't much enjoy being a tourist in my own town, but the trip does reveal a rarely seen view of my life before bringing me back to my starting point. You don't necessarily learn anything important, but you do get a fresh perspective. And that was how it was for me and my Circle Line breast cancer cruise. I couldn't help but notice some things I'd been ignoring.

Like how clueless I was about breast cancer. How susceptible to the mass media and marketers' rosy story line that keeps us all positive and optimistic and mostly quiet. I have to believe, since I certainly could have known better, that subconsciously I chose to be so uninformed because it was easier, and because, quite honestly, I never thought it would be *my* problem. Sometimes I feel kind of ashamed of my ignorance about what many breast cancer patients endure, up to and including death. I had no firsthand knowledge of it, and the message I took from the mass media was: Yeah, it's awful, but don't worry, you'll survive it.

And don't forget, we're all in this together, millions and millions of us.

I thought that was true.

But we're not all in it together. When you've marched, when you've raced, when you've worn a pink ribbon or bought a pink vacuum cleaner or blender, you've helped, but you're not in it. Not unless you know, literally all the way down into your cells, what it really means to have breast cancer.

Because if you did, you might want to do more than shop and walk for the cure. You might want to demand that more be done to learn what causes it and how to prevent it. I look at my incredible twenty-one-year-old daughter, and I want to know how she can avoid having her own diagnosis of breast cancer. I lecture her about hormones and chemicals and being vigilant, hoping that she's heard me even though she gets up and flees from the room as soon as she can. But even if she has heard me, what I'm saying isn't enough to protect her.

As the breast cancer researcher and surgeon Dr. Susan Love points out on her Web site, over the past decade two thousand breast cancer organizations have raised over $2 billion for breast cancer research, and yet we still don't know what causes it or how to prevent it, although, as Dr. Gearhart points out, tamoxifen does prevent breast cancer in some high-risk cases.

I know that breast cancer is not one simple disease, like chicken pox, with one specific cause. I know that we're getting better at finding it earlier, and that the death rate continues to go down in most categories. But I also know that the treatments that cure breast cancer can sometimes have serious side effects, like heart damage, or infertility, or lymphedema. Or other cancers. It's just not enough to treat it, we need to know what causes it.

There was a bill introduced in Congress last year that would have funded research to determine the potential links between the environment and the development of breast cancer. It would have instructed the National Institutes of Health to spend $40 million a year over the next five years. The bill had bipartisan support; it was the handiwork of the National Breast Cancer Coalition. But it was killed by Senator Tom Coburn of Oklahoma, who said he didn't want to micromanage the NIH. Coburn, a doctor, is noted for stating at a Senate hearing in 2005 that women who have silicone breast implants are actually healthier than women who don't; he's not exactly the guy I want to rely on in these matters.

It would be nice to have health care policy that wasn't politicized.

We'll Always Have October

But for now, we have Breast Cancer Awareness Month in October, and that means magazines, books, and television shows will offer a steady menu of stories about the disease for the whole month. And I do mean stories. Take it from one who used to make a very nice living producing television shows primarily for women; producers and editors are always on the lookout for compelling, inspirational breast cancer stories. Dramatic, up-close and personal sagas will nearly always trump serious (dare I say dry?), fact-based news reports unless the facts are in and of themselves dramatic—that is, a major breakthrough. There's nothing inherently evil about that, but it probably explains why, despite the heavy media attention to breast cancer, there are still so many misconceptions about the disease, and so much that the average woman could know about it but doesn't. A survey released in October 2007 by the National Breast Cancer Coalition found lots of awareness, but also lots of misunderstanding about a variety of issues, including what the risk factors are, the areas of progress, and how to try to prevent it.

And as for the news headlines we do hear about, too often they're confusing and conflicting.

It's as if there's a Newton's Law of Breast Cancer: For every breast cancer finding there is an equal and opposite breast cancer finding.

Take stress. In 2003, a study of Swedish women found that those who had stress-filled lives ran a higher risk of developing breast cancer.

Yet, in 2005, another study found that stress may actually reduce a woman's risk. Apparently, according to this study, the high-octane, pressure-cooker life associated with some careers causes a reduction in estrogen, at least among women in Copenhagen, where the study was conducted.

By the way, what do women in Sweden and Denmark have to be so damned stressed out about? Too much free health care? Too much education? Too tall and pretty?

The latest study, as I write this, is a new one showing that women whose mothers had big, rounded hips are at increased risk for breast cancer. It was a study of women born between 1934 and 1944 in Helsinki, Finland, and published in the *American Journal of Human Biology*. (All I can say is, my mother had small, narrow hips for most of her life. But Julia, if this study has merit, what can I tell you, kid?)

And then there is the constant flow of Internet stories that get e-mailed to breast cancer patients or ex-patients on a daily (hourly?) basis. I wish I had a dollar for every time I've gotten an e-mail about underwire bras or antiperspirants causing breast cancer. (They don't.) Or that red meat and alcohol cause breast cancer. (They do increase the risk.) When a new report was issued saying that, contrary to earlier theories, you increase your risk no matter what kind of alcohol you drink, whether it's hard liquor or wine, my Google news alert went into overdrive. I was inundated with stories about booze and boobs.

Maybe it's not entirely accurate, but I can't help picturing a bunch of nerdy news guys who haven't had a date in ten years just slobbering over the opportunity to file stories about hard-drinkin', dangerous women who turn out to be a danger to themselves.

Ew.

Sometimes I wish I didn't know quite so much about the news biz.

But then on the other hand, sometimes I'm very glad I do, like when I saw an upbeat press release from AstraZeneca, the makers of tamoxifen, in August of 2007, which came with the headline: BREAST CANCER SURVIVORS CARRY OPTIMISTIC OUTLOOK ON LIFE.

After cheerfully reporting that the majority of women surveyed feel that having had breast cancer made them stronger and that they're better able to put their lives in perspective, there was this:

> *Interestingly, the same survey results also suggest that there may be a "disconnect" with information regarding the chances of breast cancer returning. While the majority (78 percent) of women who have had breast cancer are concerned about recurrence, 30 percent don't believe and 23 percent aren't sure there is anything they can do to lessen the likelihood of a breast cancer recurrence and only about half (55 percent) have spoken to their doctor about recurrence.* **The survey suggests that more action and education is needed about the many ways, such as healthier eating, reducing stress and taking hormonal therapy, women can help reduce the risk of recurrence.** (Emphasis mine.)

I couldn't help but notice how artfully they'd placed the phrase "taking hormonal therapy" among the survey findings. Tamoxifen, of course, is a hormone therapy designed to prevent recurrences. It's a great drug, actually, although it's even better if you don't have a uterus and can't therefore suffer its potential side effect, which is a kind of uterine cancer. Also, it's helpful if you're not prone to blood clots or stroke, because some women who use tamoxifen suffer those very deadly side effects.

I include this press release because it's exactly the kind of information busy news editors and producers are likely to grab when they're looking to do breast cancer news stories, especially the highly prized "good news" breast cancer story.

Trouble is, it's not a news story; it just looks like one. And when those kinds of releases get picked up by the wire services or Google News, they land on the giant, steaming pile of facts, fake facts, and manufactured near-news that clutter the typical producer's computer screen. Eventually, far too many of them end up on television and in print. The fact that the information came in the form of a press release makes it a little more suspect for discerning editors, but if you're a kid in a local TV station with a news hole to fill, especially in October, this is the kind of "story" you plug right into your show rundown. That's why companies like AstraZeneca pay for surveys, after all.

It would take more than a case of breast cancer to transform me from skeptical to naïve.

That's Gonna Leave a Mark

"A really strong woman accepts the war she went through and is ennobled by her scars," said Carly Simon.

I don't feel ennobled by my scars. They are simply

another fact of my life—nothing to be proud of, nothing to be ashamed of.

Whether cancer transforms you in some way or not, it will definitely leave its mark on you, physically and emotionally. It certainly did on me. For a time during chemo, I avoided looking at myself in the mirror, naked or dressed. The boycott began when I noticed that every time I glanced at my left hand, with its constant purple bruise from the chemo IV needle, I would begin to gag. I was literally grossing myself out.

Fortunately, that phase didn't last too terribly long. Eventually, the needle pricks and bruises on my hand disappeared, and as I waited for my hair and libido to return, I found I was ready to really look at myself again.

I had a noticeable chunk removed from my right breast, a red, half-moon-shaped scar where a lymph node had been removed (it was kind of like being branded with a "c" from the Not-OK Corral), and I had an extra scar where my doctors had tried to insert the mammosite radiation device. I always imagine that particular round scar to have been caused by Dr. Hayes bracing a high heel against my rib cage as she tried to stuff the damned radiation thing into my chest. Hmm . . . maybe she should have tried that.

Any way you sliced it, so to speak, I was kind of a mess physically, and I wanted to do whatever I could to prevent another sneak attack on my health. If only I knew how.

Did Marshmallows Give Me Breast Cancer?

If only you could prevent breast cancer by changing your eating habits. Or by not smoking. Or by doing anything proactively. But as we contemplate what to do in the future, it's pretty hard not to also think about what we did in the past.

Doesn't everybody who gets cancer wonder what the hell caused it?

You don't have to have a "why me?" moment but you probably have a "what the fuck?" moment.

You're probably racking your brain, wondering what you might have breathed, eaten, smoked, rubbed on your skin, or in some other way exposed yourself to in order to trigger cancer.

It's a pointless, if unavoidable, mental exercise, because unless you're a smoker who has lung cancer or one of the other smokers' cancers, you'll probably never know.

In the months before launching Air America Radio, my colleague Lizz Winstead and I shared an office that dripped some kind of slime around the windows, and believe me, when I was diagnosed I thought about whether that crap could have caused my cells to mutate. I'll never know, but if anything looked like carcinogenic primordial ooze, it was this stuff.

I did not buy into the idea, which so many people subscribe to, that stress causes cancer. There is no serious, incontrovertible scientific evidence linking stress to breast cancer, and I have to go with science over hunches. Otherwise, I might as well be wishing on a Hope Angel.

To compensate for the fact that I'll probably never know what hit me, I'm trying to clean up my act. Literally, in some ways.

Like most, if not all, of the women I've interviewed for this book, I can honestly say that I eat better now (although some say they eat a lot more desserts, too). We eat organic foods whenever possible, and we don't eat fish full of chemicals or mercury. I never touch dairy products that were produced using hormones. And I try to avoid cosmetics that contain parabens, which mimic estrogen and just can't be good for you.

I was a big skeptic about the need for organic fabrics years ago—like, why would you need organic cotton? Who eats cotton except boll weevils?

But, in fact, cotton is one of the most heavily sprayed field crops in the world. It's just drenched in pesticides and artificial fertilizers unless it's organically grown. If I have to buy regular cotton (and I do), I at least try to wash it thoroughly before wearing it now.

There is at least one big, government-sponsored research project, the Breast Cancer and Environment Research Centers, funded by the National Institute of Environmental Health Sciences and the National Cancer Institute. One area they're studying is adolescent girls. They've found that "mounting evidence indicates that there is a window of vulnerability for breast cancer in adolescence. Environmental exposures at the time of breast development can increase the risk of breast cancer decades later."

Suddenly I flash back to my own adolescence in Omaha, and consider whether it was a bad idea to get high and stand with my nose pressed up against our family's first-generation microwave oven, watching a marshmallow expand until it was as big as the plate it was sitting on.

Damn. Did microwave marshmallows give me breast cancer?

I'm guessing not. Still, I try to be aware of everything I put in or on my body. Okay, I'll admit I still use dye to color my hair, and I still use nail polish, both of which have some evil ingredients in them, but I'm doing what I can. I have almost no booze, I take vitamins for the first time ever, and I exercise regularly.

Okay, that last part, about regular exercise, is a total lie. But I do take yoga when I can.

Surprised? Yeah, me too.

Unfinished Business

There is a term that some mental health professionals use for people who've gone through a traumatic situation and dealt with it productively. They call it post-traumatic growth syndrome (as opposed to post-traumatic stress).

I first heard the term in a yoga class created for women who'd had breast cancer.

You might well wonder what would possess a person like me to join a yoga class for women who've had breast cancer. It does seem to require me to embrace a number of activities I normally avoid, including:

A. sweating;

B. joining any sort of breast cancer group; and

C. anything that has the faintest whiff of spirituality.

But I did all three of those things when I joined the class, and while it wasn't exactly posttraumatic growth, it was some kind of a milestone. I was finally able to join a breast cancer–related group (willingly).

It all started when I noticed that I'd lost a lot of flexibility and range of motion in my right shoulder and upper arm—the side that had had the surgery. It struck me as another kind of scar, and I wanted to be rid of it, so I had taken a few private yoga classes and then ventured into some public classes, where I often made a bit of a fool of myself, but at least nobody laughed at me. I wasn't exactly a devotee like my husband, who goes to five or six classes a week, but I did enjoy the way I felt during and after class. Plus, I was starting to write this book and I knew from experience that if I didn't have some kind of exercise plan, I'd develop Author's Ass, from sitting with my laptop all day and only moving when I got up to go to the refrigerator.

At the same time, I came across a generous offer from the Libby Ross Foundation. They sponsor a number of programs for women with breast cancer, including a free yoga class at the Om Yoga center in Manhattan. Free yoga sounded good.

Joining the Club—Once a Week

I wasn't sure what it would be like to be in a group of women who were at various stages of treatment or post-treatment. It did seem, though, that it was time for me to get over myself and deal with it. What was I even afraid of? I think it was that my whole breast cancer defense system was built with tissue paper; it was possible that anybody could poke a hole in it, and then who knew what would happen? Maybe I'd discover that I wasn't the tough, impervious broad I thought I was. Maybe I'd have a retroactive freak-out and begin to live, if not in the pink bubble, at least in a closer commute to it.

On the other hand, maybe I would be just fine.

It was just yoga, just, you know, sitting in incredibly uncomfortable positions, teetering in unstable poses, breathing through my third eye, or whatever, and chanting strange syllables while trying not to seem self-conscious. What was the big deal? I decided I should not wall myself off from an experience that I might benefit from.

After all that time spent avoiding the campfires where breast cancer ghost stories were told (chat rooms, support groups, and so on), I was finally ready to hear some, now that I was at a safe distance from my own experience. I wanted to know what other women had learned and see whether it applied to me as well. And I knew I had some unfinished business with breast cancer. I had to get into a relaxed, safe place and allow myself to feel whatever emotions I'd suppressed. It wasn't a renewal of the quest for spiritual transformation so much as it was an effort to take inventory on my emotional shelves and see what was missing.

So, when the opportunity to take this yoga class presented itself, I took it.

I was a little worried about having to show some kind of proof of eligibility when I went to register. I pictured myself having to show my scar at the door. But the people at the front desk just signed me up and pointed me toward the studio. The instructors, Susan and Tari, were warm and welcoming, and about ten seconds after I walked into the class I realized that it was a great idea.

As it turned out, I became aware of my buried feelings in the very first session, as I was breathing deeply in that yoga way, and listening to our instructor talk about healing. My eyes were closed but I could feel tears spring up almost immediately behind my lids. *Whoa,* I thought. *Who knew I had so much emotion right beneath the surface?*

At any given class there may be ten women, and something less than twenty breasts. But it is so not about the breasts. Everybody is there to get back something they lost, whether it's flexibility, muscle tone, their sense of well-being, or their place in the world. Some are pale and bald, some old and determined, some heartbreakingly young and beautiful. But every one is strong. We're all there to work on ourselves, inside out.

The class was created by Tari Prinster, who'd had breast cancer herself years ago. Her class is about self-healing and self-acceptance, and what she, and others, call posttraumatic growth syndrome.

It's a syndrome I don't have, but maybe someday I will.

Tari says she began doing yoga when she was fifty, for all the wrong reasons.

"Vanity," she said, smiling. "It gave me great muscle tone, I was stronger, I had better posture. I never thought of myself as spiritual. When I got breast cancer, though, I decided I would continue to do yoga right through the treatments, every single day. It made me feel I was part of my own healing process. Everything is done to us when we have cancer, but we have to be participants."

Tari is the least judgmental woman I've ever met. I watch her sometimes out of the corner of my eye during class and wonder what's going on in her mind. But maybe the secret is what's *not* going on in her mind.

Part of my reluctance to join in any kind of breast

cancer–related community was due to the feeling that I didn't need specialized support. I've heard a lot of former breast cancer patients say they can only talk to other breast cancer survivors about it. That's never been my experience.

I have never felt that only fellow breast cancer patients could understand what I've been through. Almost everyone is capable of understanding the emotional ride of fear, pain, and feeling vulnerable—to say nothing of mortal. I assume that if you can express yourself, most people will empathize.

Still, there is a unique camaraderie in the locker room before and after breast cancer yoga class. Yoga dressing rooms are usually extremely simple affairs, no frills, just the basic storage area and benches and hooks to hang your clothes on, and this one is no different. But as we dress and chat and compare notes, some things are definitely different. I can remember racing into the dressing room, late, before a class, and struggling to get into a jogging bra that was twisted and sticking to my sweaty back. A yoga classmate whom I knew just a little bit offered to help, and got it straightened out for me.

In this socially awkward situation I attempted some small talk. I asked her if she bothered with a workout bra for yoga class.

"My breasts are here," she said, holding up a gym bag. I gasped, and tried to stammer something, an apology, or . . .

And then she giggled, allowing me to laugh at myself,

and my cluelessness. Two years after breast cancer, I was still a newbie about a lot of things.

Sometimes the dressing room fills up with women for the next (regular people) yoga class, and I can't help but notice some of them straining to hear our conversations, wanting to know, but not wanting to know. I get it; I'd do the same thing.

I also occasionally work out at a regular gym. And I've noticed an unexpected benefit from having had breast cancer—the absolutely only one I can find, but at least it's something.

You know how some women will walk around the locker room totally naked after a workout and a shower? They'll sit bare-assed on a stool blow-drying their hair, they'll rub moisturizing cream over their whole bodies in front of everybody, they'll have long conversations with their babysitters, wearing nothing but their cell phones.

I was never one of those chicks, not even in my thin years. I was always more the wrap-a-towel-around-your-body-and-get-dressed-as-fast-as-possible type. Anything to prevent someone from looking at my dimpled butt.

But now, since my lumpectomy, problem solved! My breast is just enough of a scarred-up curiosity, especially when I raise my arm over my head while getting dressed, that it distracts attention from my ass. The silent, knowing stares from across the locker room now are prompted by sympathy instead of disdain. It's a beautiful thing.

There—see? I was able to find some happy talk about breast cancer after all.

A Lesson Not Learned from Breast Cancer

"It's important to be participants in our healing. We can have a lot of control. I hired a friend to come over while I was in treatment to teach me how to do positive meditation, which helped a lot with anxiety. That was a big gift to myself. What made me healthy was to be treated as normal, as a strong and healthy woman, not as a freak or a fragile creature."

—Tari Prinster, yoga instructor

Chapter Nine

Pink Isn't Black or White

We Shop. Therefore We Cure.

The number-one killer of women is not breast cancer. It's not lung cancer, either (although lung cancer is the number-one cancer killer of women in America). The number-one killer of women, overall, is heart disease. Heart disease kills *ten times* more women every year than breast cancer.

I guess I was dimly aware that February is Heart Disease Awareness Month, and that its color is red, like valentines and hearts that aren't covered in sticky, gooey, killer plaque. But that's about all I knew. I didn't know, for example, that the heart disease symbol for women is a pin shaped like a red dress, a sexy, capped-sleeved number with a scooped neckline. Personally, I'd say if you can wear a hot little red dress like that without fear of exposing a pair of flapping bingo wings, you probably aren't at high risk for a heart attack, but maybe that's just me showing my ignorance.

Maybe that's just me saying to myself, wow, the fashion industry came up with this dress symbol, and it's sort of designed for skinny models, and wouldn't many of them drastically lower their risk of heart attack if they'd just stop snorting cocaine and smoking cigarettes for dinner?

Maybe the red dress pin is just another example of the American consumer economy trying to deal with a serious medical problem by appealing to what they perceive is every woman's passion for fashion.

(Do they not see how we actually dress most of the time? Could they not design a pin shaped like red sweatpants, or skintight red jeans with muffin tops hanging over the waistband?)

And while we're talking about Heart Awareness Month, did you know there is a National Wear Red Day in February? I didn't, either, but once I heard about it and went to shop for something red to show my, um, awareness, the choices were shockingly limited. Not like, you know, breast cancer. No wonder we don't know as much as we need to about our heart health. I mean, like, where's the merch? Compared to breast cancer's online malls, the choices on the heart health awareness Web sites are kind of sad.

Come on, people, there are lives at stake here.

All kidding aside, I'm not singling out the Go Red for Women campaign. It takes time for awareness campaigns to grow and they haven't been at it for more than a few years. But it does make you wonder if every public health education campaign these days has to come with a full array of awareness and support tchotchkes.

There are so many Web sites offering pins, buttons, rubber bracelets, baseball caps, teddy bears, and so on, I can't even name them all. Do they all donate proceeds from their sales to the disease charities for which they're promoting awareness? The ones I queried said they did, but I'd have no way of knowing whether they really do, and if so, to which charities, and how much, unless I did an awful lot of digging. I imagine they depend more on impulse buying than on smart consumerism.

One of the largest Web sites, which says it contributes every year to more than twenty charities but doesn't list which ones or say how much they give, sells a staggering array of "awareness" items, from "The Power of Hope" bracelets to breast cancer cookie cutters (which are shaped like pink ribbons, not, as I feared for a fleeting moment, tumors). And, of course, there are "huggables," which are stuffed dogs and teddy bears that have names. And there's even a Pillow of Hope.

What's with all the "hope" stuff, anyway? "Wishin' and Hopin'" didn't help the late Dusty Springfield at all when she had breast cancer. Of course I believe in hope (I have hope every time I try on a bathing suit, let alone when I'm waiting for test results), but hope as a cancer strategy seems awfully old-school passive to me. Even if some portion of the money you spend on "hope" goes directly to research, it rubs me the wrong way. I consider "hope" to be the catalyst for action, not the action itself.

I am not doubting the sincerity of the people behind these online breast cancer pinkatoriums, although you could make the argument that sites that just sell stuff, and include no educational information, are exploiting women with the disease and trivializing the breast cancer awareness movement. And I'm not doubting the sincerity of the people who buy things either for themselves or a friend. Whatever gets you through the night—angels, elves, huggables, bracelets—if it makes you feel better, go for it.

But I can't help it if I find some of this stuff kind of, let's just say, over the top. And it's not just for breast cancer.

Take, for example, the Web site www.choosehope.com. (There's that word again.) They "offer a full line of cancer gifts for you and your family . . . If you or someone you know has just been diagnosed, this is the site for you!" So, if you've "just been diagnosed," don't even bother visiting a Web site that can tell you more about your disease—not until you've been to choosehope.com. What are you, some kind of cancer nerd? Choose Hope tells us it was created by women who had breast cancer. You might expect, therefore, that they would think twice before selling a button that proclaims, "Colon Cancer Can be a Real Pain in the Butt."

Ya think? And yes, that is an actual button for sale on their Web site as I write this. And all you lymphoma patients, be sure to check out that "I'm a Lymphomaniac" button. If laughter is the best medicine, why, you'll be cured in no time!

Oh, wait, no, you won't, because that's not funny.

Of course there are other Web sites offering a selection

of buttons, bracelets, and ribbons, too, like personalized-cause.com. There you can buy a ribbon for virtually any-thing that ails you, like, say, acid reflux. The acid reflux ribbon, which I would have thought would be a bilious yel-low, happens to be periwinkle blue. Not to make fun of people who have acid reflux, which I know can be painful and burn the esophagus, but do we really need to build awareness for a disease that can be treated with TUMS? Should there be a Race for the Rolaids?

If you want to build awareness for agoraphobia, the rib-bon is a lovely shade of teal. Hey, wait a minute; agorapho-bics don't even *go* shopping. They don't go anywhere. They're agoraphobic! So who will see their ribbons and become aware?

On the other hand, if chemo's got you bald, you might show your solidarity with alopecia survivors, by picking up a blue rubber "Know More" wristband.

Both personalizedcause.com and choosehope.com re-sponded to my e-mail queries by telling me that profits from some of their sales do go to charity, but they were not specific about how much. Choosehope.com does list the charities it says it contributes to, and seems to have a monthly $5,000 donation to one of them, which is good to know.

It is extraordinary that we've all come to believe that the best way to donate money is to buy things we don't need, rather than giving it directly to the charity we want to help. But millions and millions of dollars get raised that way for breast cancer, so obviously it's a very successful strategy.

Actually, I shouldn't be surprised. After all, we are a nation that was told after 9/11 that we could all do our part in the war on terrorism by resuming our shopping ("continued participation in our economy" was the actual phrase).

In some countries, when there is a horrible problem affecting one-third of the population, the citizens vote for leaders whom they believe will make policies to deal with that problem. But in America, Land of Too Much Everything, where one in three citizens will develop some kind of cancer in his or her lifetime, what we do to affect public policy is shop. It's nice to buy things, but it's not a substitute for action.

The Web sites offering awareness-abilia for whatever disease you can imagine, and some you cannot, are clearly trying to repeat the success of the breast cancer awareness movement.

But that success didn't happen overnight or by accident. Breast cancer as a cause had to fight its way to center stage, and it got there not because of ladies who shop, but thanks to women who lobby. It took almost thirty years for breast cancer to become corporate America's sweetheart charity. Travel back with me, if you will, to the beginning of the modern breast cancer awareness movement, in the 1970s.

From the Disease That Dares Not Speak Its Name to the Disease That Everybody's Talking About

The '70s were a transitional time in our society—Morning After in America. The social change that began in the '60s with the baby boomers' simple, modestly expressed desire, "We want the world and we want it now," led to rather more specific, grown-up demands, such as equal rights for women. The draft-card-burning hippies were joined by the (mythical) bra-burning women's libbers as the scary symbols of social revolution.

Still, almost nobody was untouched by the social changes of the times, not even good Republican wives. So it was that as feminists were powering the women's health movement, their demands for better breast cancer care were helped considerably by a Nixon appointee, the former actress Shirley Temple Black, as well as by Betty Ford and Happy Rockefeller.

Because she was First Lady at the time of her diagnosis, Betty Ford's breast cancer got most of the media attention. She got a lot of credit for being so forthright about the disease, but she wasn't the first famous woman to shatter the conventions of polite society by using both the words "breast" and "cancer" out loud.

Two years earlier, in 1972, America's favorite child star, Shirley Temple Black, found a lump in her breast during a routine self-exam. She chose to go public with her whole story, according to *Bathsheba's Breast*, "for all of my sisters who have lost a breast, for all of my sisters who fear they may."

What was equally impressive to me is that Ms. Black did her own research, decades before the Internet, and decided that she would not undergo the one-step surgery that was standard operating procedure. At the time, nearly all women suspected of having breast cancer went into the hospital for a biopsy, and while they were under anesthesia, their doctors would check for cancer. If they found it, the women woke up without a breast.

Several years later, the breast cancer advocate Rose Kushner led a successful movement to stop "one-step mastectomies," but Shirley Temple Black was ahead of her time. "The doctor will make the incision, I'll make the decision," she's quoted as saying in *Bathsheba's Breast*.

And, on top of that, she knew enough to insist that a radical mastectomy was not necessary, and searched until she found doctors who agreed to do a simple mastectomy.

She wrote about her experience in an article for *McCall's* magazine; and thus was born a new genre in women's media: the personal breast cancer story.

I confess those early breast cancer stories didn't have much of an impact on my life back then; the women's health issues of concern to me were reproductive rights. I thought I was too young to think about breast cancer, believing incorrectly that it was a disease that only struck older women. My mother and her peers weren't even at prime risk age yet, and I didn't know anybody who'd had it. No doubt the newsrooms of America, with their nearly all-male staffs, had little or no interest in assigning stories about breast cancer except when a famous woman had it. Mostly it was the stuff of women's pages and women's magazines.

Luckily, breast cancer advocates didn't wait for men to get over their embarrassment.

Breast cancer has evolved from the disease that dare not speak its name to the disease that everybody talks about. Some frustrated activists for other causes say it's also the disease that doesn't allow anybody else to get a word in edgewise. They may be frustrated, but breast cancer advocacy is a classic example of a grassroots movement powered by highly motivated women who earned their place of respect in the public consciousness and political agenda. They are the role model to follow; but they had a role model once, too.

In the Beginning There Was the Ribbon, and It Was Red

The pink ribbon is directly descended from the red ribbon of the HIV/AIDS movement. In 1991, artist-activists in a group called Visual AIDS came up with the red ribbon in response to the yellow ribbons that commemorated

American soldiers fighting in the Gulf War. Men were dying in America, too, of AIDS, and the artists in Visual AIDS wanted to create a symbolic reminder of that. The red ribbon was first worn publicly by Jeremy Irons at the 1991 Tony Awards. Months later, pink ribbons were distributed at a Komen race for the cure in New York. In October 1992, *Self* magazine and Evelyn Lauder began distributing pink ribbons for breast cancer awareness nationally.

There were other ways that breast cancer activists followed in the footsteps of the AIDS activism movement. They began to organize to lobby and demand more federal funding for breast cancer research and more affordable health care. The group Y-ME was formed in Chicago, and one of its founders, Sheila Swanson, told the *New York Times* back then that AIDS activists "showed us how to get through to the government. They took an archaic system and turned it around while we have been quietly dying." (Interestingly, AIDS activists credit the feminists who started the women's health movement as their original role models.) The National Breast Cancer Coalition (NBCC) was also created that year. As a Washington-based organization, the NBCC lobbied Congress for more funding, and their activism paid off.

At the time, the federal government was spending a little over a billion dollars on AIDS research and about $77 million on breast cancer. By contrast, in 2007, the National Cancer Institute alone was budgeted to spend $551 million on breast cancer, and total government funding on breast cancer will be nearly a billion dollars.

The organizations like the National Breast Cancer Coalition did an incredible job organizing, lobbying, and educating volunteers so that they, too, could become advocates. They pushed hard to get "civilians" on policy-making boards so they could have input as research priorities were set.

Of course it helped that breast cancer was a completely noncontroversial way to deal with a women's policy issue. Unlike abortion or birth control, unlike equal rights in the workplace and in publicly funded education, there really was only one side in the breast cancer discussion. And best of all for politicians, it was a disease that had nothing to do with behavior or bad habits. It wasn't like lung cancer, or AIDS, or heart disease. You couldn't just make a lifestyle adjustment to improve your chances of avoiding it. If someone's mother or wife or sister got breast cancer, it wasn't "her fault."

And the epidemic was growing worse; there were so many, many mothers and wives and sisters who were getting the disease.

But that only partly explains how the breast cancer movement evolved into the pinkapalooza it is today.

What started as a three-pronged attack to defeat breast cancer—one political, one medical, and one social—has morphed into a situation where everybody uses everybody. Mostly it's for the same worthy goal—ending breast cancer.

But, hey, the drug companies can't help it if there's also a tidy profit in it for them, can they?

And Now a Word from Our Sponsors

It's hard to remember an October that wasn't Breast Cancer Awareness Month. In fact, the first BCAM was in 1985, and its cocreator and major sponsor was, and continues to be, AstraZeneca, the makers of tamoxifen and a newer hormone therapy, Arimidex. Now, you could be cynical and say to yourself, "Gosh, that means that the people who are telling women to get an annual mammogram are in effect drumming up new business for themselves. More women diagnosed with breast cancer means more women buying tamoxifen means more profits for AstraZeneca."

Just ask Michael Zubillaga, a regional sales director for AstraZeneca, who was quoted in the *Oncology* newsletter as saying this about doctors' offices, according to *Brandweek* and other news outlets:

"There is a big bucket of money sitting in every office. Every time you go in, you reach your hand in the bucket and grab a handful. The more times you are in, the more money goes in your pocket."

On second thought, don't ask him. He got fired for that and other comments.

Do you ever get the feeling that you may call yourself

a survivor, but the drug companies call you a customer? Yeah, me too.

By the way, it's not just breast cancer drugs; that Go Red for Women heart awareness campaign is cosponsored by Merck, which makes the cholesterol-lowering drug Zocor. Sure, it's possible that Merck simply has women's heart health in mind and isn't looking to whip up business by encouraging women to find out if they have high cholesterol and therefore might become Zocor users. But I think it's safe to assume that they want to be associated with a good cause that generates profits. And that is what is known as cause marketing, which has been honed to an art form by the Pink Ribbonistas.

The Rise of Cause Marketing

The pharmaceutical industry is sometimes accused of "disease marketing," which is basically what happens when suddenly you learn, through advertising, of the likelihood that you have a condition, a disease, or a syndrome (restless leg, anyone?) for which a drug company just happens to have a new cure. Drug company creates need, consumer responds by buying product to meet that need. It's the American way. The transaction is pretty straightforward.

The same cannot be said of the marketing tactic that is responsible for so many of the pink ribbon products for sale during Breast Cancer Awareness Month and beyond. When a big consumer brand pledges that part of the proceeds of whatever product it's selling will go to a charity, that's a strategy known as cause marketing. It's a common practice now for corporations to attach themselves to worthy causes, selling their products while at the same time buying good-will. American Express is considered the first corporation to use cause-related marketing; in 1983 the company donated a penny from every Amex card purchase to the fund to re-furbish the Statue of Liberty. Now, nobody does it better than breast cancer advocates like the Susan G. Komen for the Cure Foundation and the Breast Cancer Research Foun-dation.

It's a trend that worries professionals in the charitable fund-raising world. I had an interesting conversation with Sandra Miniutti, of the Web site charitynavigator.org, which tracks how charities spend the money they take in.

"Cause marketing has taken off most dramatically for breast cancer," she told me. "In October you can't go any-where without buying a pink ribbon. I think this is partly because Komen has led the way, from KitchenAid to BMW, and they've done an amazing job. But on the negative side, for consumers it's very difficult to understand how much money gets to the charity. It could be only cents on the dol-lar really going to the charity. It may be that companies are donating only on the first hundred products sold, and then none of the rest. Corporations can set a ceiling on how much money is going to the charity."

The very-high-end jeweler Cartier provided an example of that a couple of years ago. Cartier sold a pink watch for $3,900 and promised to donate $30,000 to the Breast Cancer Research Foundation. So, if you were the ninth or tenth woman to buy that watch, all of your money went to the nice people at Cartier, and not a penny of it went to breast cancer research. After taking some heat, Cartier changed its policy, and announced the next year that it was donating $200 per sale, with a minimum of $16,000.

Sandra explained why the charities and the corporations find cause-related marketing to be so attractive.

"Charities get access to a marketing and advertising budget in amounts they'd never normally have access to, which hopefully generates revenue for them. The corporation is borrowing the image of the charity, using it to sell their products and services."

But why breast cancer? I asked. Why not heart disease or prostate cancer?

"Breast cancer was just out there first with cause-related marketing and beat the other causes to the punch," she replied. "I also think people are much more stricken when they hear about a mother, a young woman, or someone we know who has breast cancer.

"Other causes have tried to duplicate what breast cancer has accomplished, like Lance Armstrong and his LIVE-STRONG bracelet, and Bono with the Red campaign, but nobody has yet been as successful."

If you participate in the pinkapalooza, do your homework

and read the fine print. You may be buying pink stuff you really didn't want, and be failing to contribute anything to fighting breast cancer.

Charitynavigator.org is one good resource—they rate the charities on criteria like how much money gets directly to the recipients, and how efficient the charity is in terms of administrative and fund-raising costs. By their standards, Komen gets four stars, as does Y-ME, Living Beyond Breast Cancer, and the National Breast Cancer Research Foundation, which is the organization founded by Evelyn Lauder of the Estée Lauder cosmetics family. There are others that rank as high, and some that do far less well.

A survey done in 2007 for the cause-marketing industry found that 87 percent of American consumers say they would switch from one brand to another if the other brand were associated with a good cause.

So I think you can expect to see more pink blenders and vacuum cleaners and lawn mowers in the future. But, please—no more Pink Ribbon Barbies.

Cash Cow Barbie to the Rescue

In the context of what it's really like to have suffered the trauma of this disease, and to continue to live with its impact on our physical and emotional health, our sexuality, and our outlook on life, you can probably imagine the reaction generated by the news that Mattel was rolling out Pink Ribbon Barbie.

On blogs all over the Internet, angry breast cancer patients railed against the insensitivity of promoting Barbie, plastic princess of perky tits, as a new symbol of "breast cancer awareness." Using *the* retro icon of the unattainable beauty standard of our youth—huge, high breasts, tiny waist, no butt, and long, slim, undimpled thighs—to help women with breast cancer? Pretty hilarious.

Breast cancer patients reacted with predictable snark and sarcasm on blogs and messages boards from coast to coast.

"Why does she still have two breasts?"

"Why isn't she bald?"

"Where's the little pink toilet for when she needs to puke?"

And on and on.

Other women defended Pink Ribbon Barbie as a lovely way to remind themselves to get their annual mammograms. I would have thought Pink Ribbon PalmPilot, or Pink Ribbon desk calendar would have worked as well, but, hey, what do I know?

I do worry about those women, though; if they cling to Barbie as their style and beauty role model, I'd imagine they'll have a hell of a time if they ever do lose a breast to cancer someday.

I suppose if adult women need Barbie dolls to remember to get mammograms, that's okay. But, with all due respect,

Mattel, it's hard to believe that the average breast cancer patient is going to be all that excited by the news that Barbie is "stylishly joining the fight against breast cancer," with her shiny hair cascading down her shoulders and her big tits filling out a "frothy pink organza gown featuring a shirred design and tiers of ruffles." How is Barbie fighting breast cancer, anyway? Well, clearly she's working the streets, or at least the toy shelves, for Mattel, with some of the proceeds going to Komen. But that's not all she's doing, bless her heart.

The press release announcing the doll helpfully points out that Pink Ribbon Barbie "can serve as a communication vehicle to open a dialogue about breast cancer with children."

Really?

How does that dialogue go?

Maybe like this:

"Kids, see this Barbie? This is what Mommy never looked like. And now that she's got breast cancer, she doesn't look like Barbie even more."

As far as the fund-raising ability of cash cow Barbie, well, thanks for all that, Mattel, but you could just write a freaking check to breast cancer research. Something is always better than nothing, but $2.50 per $25 sale, with a guaranteed minimum check of $100,000 to Susan G. Komen, is not all that impressive.

Barbie was created by Ruth Handler, who maintained

that the doll's huge breasts would be good for the self-esteem of young girls unsure about their developing bodies.

Barbie was probably the gateway ~~drug~~ toy to a future of distorted body-image issues for me. But I'm not bitter. Really.

I got my first Barbie when I was about seven. She was clearly an aspirational doll, although we didn't have terms like "aspirational" back then. She was blonde, she had blue eyes, she had giant boobs and a tiny waist. I was short, I had brown hair and eyes, I had a giant waist and no boobs. She was a fairy princess, I was the little brown toad who gets ditched by the bigger brown toad after a princess kisses him and turns him into a prince. Still, I loved Barbie, from the moment I saw her in her strange zebra-striped strapless bathing suit with her open-toed, high-heeled mules. It wasn't weird to me that her earrings were pearls on a pin that you stuck straight into her plastic head. But there was one weird thing about Barbie.

She didn't make eye contact with you. She would not return your worshipful gaze. The early Barbies' eyes were all created to look away, as if they were scoping out the room for some hottie to go over and flirt with. It was like being rejected by your own doll. Barbie as Mean Girl.

"Yeah, yeah, dress me. Whatever. Don't you know any cute guys?" she seemed to be saying.

Well, no, I don't, but, hey, look, Barbie, I bought you the great cocktail dress with the red velveteen bodice and the full white satin skirt from the catalogue. See? If you'd just look in my direction . . . I'd say to her silently. But no. There was no pleasing the heartless bitch.

Screw it then, Barbie, I'm going to dress you in the red sweater and skirt outfit my grandmother knitted for you that I had to pretend I liked. Yeah, you're right, you do look like a librarian. And Ken's coming over. No, I won't put you back in your toreador pants and halter top.

Like I said, I'm not bitter.

Having made jokes at the expense of Pink Ribbon Barbie and the various online pinkatoriums, I must add that I know cause marketing works. It's raised hundreds of millions of dollars for breast cancer research. I'm sure that's what is so maddening to the women who complain that it's nothing but corporate exploitation of breast cancer. But do we really want to jeopardize the pink ribbon awareness campaigns' unbelievable track record for fund-raising? I don't, although I wish there were an equally effective alternative.

Nobody speaks more passionately about the shortcomings of the cause-marketing campaigns than the "Bad Girls of Breast Cancer," as the group Breast Cancer Action is called. In their "Think Before You Pink" campaign, they point out that some corporate sponsors are themselves guilty of using or manufacturing potentially carcinogenic chemicals in their products, so that their sponsorship of breast cancer awareness is "pink washing."

Breast Cancer Action (and others) also argue that the

hundreds of millions of dollars pouring into breast cancer research are not well coordinated, often are used to duplicate work done by others, and are not adequately spent on searching for the causes of the disease. I agree.

Still, if people didn't choose to donate to their favorite charity by spending all that money on pink ribbon stuff, corporations wouldn't do cause marketing. In this country we have a bake-sale philosophy of fund-raising for national crises. Don't just ask for money, get a third party to put up some product (like, say, you, baking brownies), which you then sell to people who otherwise might not have dropped a dollar into the kitty. It's easier to pass up a collection basket than a plate full of brownies.

How Much Awareness Is Enough?

Another argument made by the critics of pink ribbon awareness campaigns is that we don't need to raise awareness anymore. They say it's time for action, not awareness. While it is certainly time for action, there are still some issues with awareness.

For one, the number of women who get annual mammograms is actually decreasing. In the year 2000, 70 percent of women forty years old or older reported having a mammogram recently, but in 2005 the number fell to 66 percent. Even worse, the dropoff was greatest among women aged fifty to sixty-four, probably the age group that would benefit most from yearly mammograms. (This comes from a federally funded National Health Interview Study.) Nobody knows why the change occurred, but the authors of the study theorize some possible reasons are higher costs, less access, and less perceived risk of dying from breast cancer.

The lead research analyst told the *Washington Post*, "Women may also be feeling, 'Well, the death rates are dropping in the population so I don't need to get screened.' . . . That's kind of missing the point. One reason death rates are dropping is because screening rates were so high."

There are still segments of the population who have never been screened, either because they have no access to appropriate health care or because they come from communities that have a "don't ask, don't tell" attitude about breast cancer, for social or cultural reasons.

Young breast cancer patients often say they didn't know as much as they might have, because for all the "awareness" talk in October, we don't do a good job of educating young women about risk factors for their age group.

And for all the years of "awareness" campaigns, how many women are aware of a kind of breast cancer that does not present itself with a lump? It's called inflammatory breast cancer (IBC), and if you've never heard of this, you're not alone. It's very aggressive, but fortunately, rare. It's caused when cancer cells block lymph vessels in the breast, making the breast look "inflamed" and often red and swollen.

It's often misdiagnosed as an infection at first—there are many doctors who've never seen a case of inflammatory breast cancer so they don't recognize it. And sadly, the five-year survival rate for IBC is only between 25 and 50 percent. It's treated with pretty much everything medicine can throw at it: chemotherapy, surgery, radiation, and hormone therapy, and they are making progress—there are better treatments, so there is hope, but it's a long, rough road.

According to the National Cancer Institute, 1 to 5 percent of breast cancer patients have IBC. That sounds like a small number, but when you consider that in 2007 an estimated 178,000 women in America were diagnosed with breast cancer, we're still talking about thousands of women having this awful strain of the disease that many of us have barely heard of.

There is far too much that we aren't aware of to declare Breast Cancer Awareness Month obsolete or unnecessary. And while I hate the fact that October has become the catchall time for breast cancer coverage, at least that month prompts news organizations to look for, and present, informative stories about it.

If your way of promoting awareness is to buy pink tchotchkes, you owe it to yourself, and the people you want to help, to "think before you pink," as Breast Cancer Action says.

All of the major breast cancer charitable foundations recommend you ask a series of questions, including: Does the brand have a history of commitment to the cause it is promoting? How much of the money spent by the consumer gets to the charity? How reputable is the charity? How does the charity spend its money?

Breast Cancer Action also wants you to go further—asking whether the company whose product you're considering can assure you that its products do not contribute to the breast cancer epidemic through pollution or potentially carcinogenic ingredients. Plus, know which charity the product is contributing to, and what kind of research or support the organization is helping to fund.

Or you could do something crazy, like choosing your favorite breast cancer charity and sending them a check.

This is a chapter largely about the marketing of a public health crisis. But we haven't talked about the most powerful marketing tool of all: fear.

Be Afraid. Be Very Afraid. But Maybe Not *That* Afraid.

Remember when America was the land of the free and the home of the brave? When freedom from fear was considered a fundamental right of every American, as Franklin Roosevelt declared in his Four Freedoms speech in 1941? Turns out, when we're healthy and safe and have nothing much to be afraid of, we crave fear; we're junkies for it. When we're not actually threatened, fear entertains us, it informs us, it motivates us. Fear is for sale every day in this country, in books and movies and TV shows, in political campaigns ("If you vote for him, America is going to get hit again"), in public health crusades. Fear replaces thoughtful debate and careful, considered policy making—fear translates to "do it or else."

And I would have to say fear is used as a motivational tool in the fight against breast cancer. Which is too bad.

In order to convince women to get an annual mammogram, the breast cancerocracy informs us that one in eight of us will get breast cancer. That is a terrifying statistic. It's also more than a little bit misleading; the fact is, what that statistic actually means is that one in eight women who live to be eighty-five (some say ninety-five) will get breast cancer in their lifetimes. It's much more effective—meaning scarier—to allow women of all ages to believe their chances are one in eight. In fact, a woman between the ages of forty and forty-nine has a 1 in 68 chance, and a woman between thirty and thirty-nine has a 1 in 229 chance of having breast cancer. (These are statistics from the National Cancer Institute.)

Don't get me wrong; I believe we should all have annual mammograms. I don't know where I'd be today if not for a mammogram. But I didn't go for it because I was afraid I'd be one of eight who'd get breast cancer; I went because I understood it was part of basic health care maintenance, one of many things I do to try to stay healthy.

Remember the documentary called *Scared Straight?* It came out in 1978, and won an Oscar. The whole idea was to take some juvenile offenders, plop them down in Rahway State Prison in New Jersey, and let the inmates scream at them and intimidate them about how awful prison life is until the kids were scared straight. Yes, that extreme tactic worked, but most kids don't need to face down a crew of hard-guy inmates to understand that it's wrong to break the law. And I suspect that most women don't need to be threatened with cancer to understand that it's wise to have regular checkups, including mammograms.

(Although . . . imagine for a moment if a bunch of women who hadn't been diligent about getting mammograms were shipped off to a breast cancer support group and made to sit there while half a dozen hardened breast cancer patients screamed at them about what their daily lives were like? I know . . . we could call it Scared Squished.)

Some of us probably do need a kick in the butt, but I for one would welcome seeing women treated like adults, or at least like recovering fear junkies, because fear makes us powerless; it infantilizes us.

Honestly, couldn't we just this once have an appropriate public education campaign, with or without pink huggables and ribbons, to convince women that, like going to the dentist or the gynecologist for routine health care, they need to have their breasts checked once a year?

The larger problem with fear tactics is that they only tell part of the story and we need to hear all of it. Sounding the alarm is one thing—but it's only one thing. Make me aware of the potential danger, yes, please. But don't stop there. And don't try to lull me into thinking that if I do this thing, I've protected myself. Don't tell us that mammograms are our best defense against breast cancer. They don't defend us against an attack; they only reveal that one has happened.

I would dress in pink from head to toe every day if it would bring real awareness, or even begin a serious national dialogue on the causes and prevention of cancer for everybody.

But what I won't do is get caught up in fear-based, rather than science-based, marketing tactics.

The Few, the Scared, the Targeted: The BRCA Gene Test Ads

If you live in the northeast, you may have seen a commercial that urges women to find out whether they have the BRCA 1 or 2 gene mutation that so often leads to breast cancer. The ad recommends testing, and gives a toll-free number to call for more information. You have to pay attention to the fine print at the end to discover that the ad is sponsored by the very company that conducts the gene testing, so it is safe to assume that the company, Myriad Genetics, is running this ad for the same reason all for-profit companies run ads—to drum up business, not merely to perform a public service by "raising public awareness," as the company proclaims. What they don't tell you in the commercial is that the risk that you have the gene mutation is about 1 in 400, or one-quarter of 1 percent, and that the test costs more than $3,000. (Women of Ashkenazi Jewish descent have a higher risk, and because scientists have isolated the part of the gene that needs to be tested on those women—I'm one of them—their cost of being tested is much less.)

The goal of this ad is to urge (scare) women into calling their doctors to demand that they be tested, despite the remote possibility that they have the gene mutation. A governmental advisory group suggested that about 2 percent of women are reasonable candidates for the test. Myriad Genetics, I would assume, would not be happy with the profit potential on testing just 2 percent of customers.

And by the way, the BRCA gene mutations are responsible for only about 5 to 10 percent of all breast cancer cases.

Just once I'd like to see a commercial that ends with, "Ask your doctor if vodka is right for you."

A Lesson Not Learned from Breast Cancer

"The bottom line is I don't think I learned anything from breast cancer—except that I hope it never comes back. I didn't need to have breast cancer to learn about me or life. It did confirm some things I was already pretty sure were true, the best thing being that my husband is truly a wonderful human being and I really did marry the right guy! And that my kids are resilient and good people. Also, all my friends really are my friends—no one let me down."

—Fiona Conway

Chapter Ten

Why I Don't Call Myself a Survivor

The term "cancer survivor" was coined in 1986 by an organization called the National Coalition for Cancer Survivorship, a committed and dedicated advocacy group. They define the term this way: "From the moment of diagnosis and for the balance of life, an individual diagnosed with cancer is a survivor." That definition was ultimately adopted by most of the cancer community.

The goal back then was to empower people with cancer to become more assertive and knowledgeable about their own health care and to push for increased funding for research. Obviously that was a good thing, although I do quibble with the later inclusion of loved ones and other caregivers as "survivors."

Actually, I quibble with the whole definition.

If you're a survivor the day you find out you have a disease, doesn't it sound a little like you're declaring yourself a winner at the very beginning of the game? Don't you have to play the game—or have the treatment—before saying you've defeated your adversary?

Are you a winner if you just made the team, especially if you didn't even have to try out for it?

I Know You Are but What Am I?

I do not call myself a survivor. That's my personal choice; I know that's probably the word you use to describe yourself, and that's fine by me. I don't want to rain on anybody's parade. I think most people who use that term do so because it makes them feel strong and victorious. But for me, not so much. For one thing, to the extent possible, I want to resist labeling myself in terms of cancer, and I know a fair number of other women who feel the same way.

But mainly, it would make me a little nervous to call myself a survivor. To me, "survivor" is a term for someone who has

A. had a serious brush with death, and
B. escaped it.

Both of those conditions have to be met in my definition. By those standards, I can't call myself a survivor.

Take part one: I didn't see myself as having an actual brush with death. It was more like Death sent me a post-card with the words "Thinking of You" inscribed on it. It was kind of a spooky reminder that Death is out there somewhere, but it was not exactly a brush, per se. I never saw myself as being at Death's door. And I certainly never thought Death was at my doorstep, although if he was wearing a red-striped shirt and carrying a pizza box my doorman would wave him right through to my apartment.

And then there's part two: Let's just say, for argument's sake, that it *was* a brush with death. I can't guarantee that I've escaped it forever.

I mean, if you were in a plane crash and you walked away from it unhurt, it can't come back to harm you later. Hence, you are a plane crash survivor, most definitely.

Now, if you have another plane crash, a recurrence, if you will, and you walk away from that one, too, I guess you could say you're a two-time survivor, but I would suggest you find some other means of transportation. And remind me never to fly with you.

Breast cancer is not in any way like being in a plane crash, and I'm just not sure I can ever call myself a survivor, in the traditional sense of the word. With breast cancer, you can be clean for years—in essence, walk away from the crash—and then get it again. That's the thing about breast cancer. If you go five years your odds are good, but you're never totally in the clear. You can get a recurrence any old time, or you may be cured of one breast cancer, but get a completely new, unrelated one. Fran Visco, president of the National Breast Cancer Coalition (NBCC), told the *New York Times* that "you are never assured that the disease will not come back." The NBCC uses the term, "but only because most people accept it."

To me, the answer to the question, "Well, then how do you know if you're really cured of breast cancer?" is, "When you die of something else."

So, if I was walking down the street to cash in a winning ticket for the million-dollar lottery and a grand piano dropped out of the sky and squashed me flat, my family could say I was a breast cancer survivor who got killed by a grand piano.

And had very mixed luck.

I'm not willing to tempt fate. I will watch out for falling grand pianos, but I just won't call myself a breast cancer survivor.

I guess that makes me a very odd combination of superstitious and realistic at the same time.

And by the way, did you ever wonder why it is that cancer, alone among illnesses, is something that you are a survivor of as soon as you know you have it? We chuckle a little to hear that forty years ago, doctors didn't tell patients they had cancer, because they thought they couldn't handle it. But telling cancer patients they are survivors the minute they're diagnosed just feels like a more modern version of the same verbal obfuscation to me, a way of avoiding the term "cancer" and choosing instead a more positive, upbeat word. Maybe it's just their version of denial.

I know this is a loaded topic—words matter to all of us—but I've thought about it a lot and this is how I come out on "survivor" in terms of me. I would also point out that the group that coined the term, the NCCS, says "it is descriptive, it's not meant to be biologically correct."

Here's what else I won't call myself:

I am not a soldier. I'm not a warrior. Breast cancer reminded me that I loathe military metaphors, because I think they trivialize the true, unremitting hell of warfare.

Pink is not the new camouflage.

I did not "battle" breast cancer. I hosted a chemical and radiological assault conducted on my behalf, on territory that happens to be my body, but it wasn't a war. Hell, I didn't even know I'd been attacked until doctors told me.

Talk about living with "sleeper cells."

From June of 2004 to February of 2005, while I was being forced to host my treatments, I hunkered down. I tried to carry on with my life and live as normally as possible, like one of those brave women in real war zones who dodge snipers' bullets and land mines to go out and forage some food for their children. But my breast cancer treatment was never that terrifying. In my case, the only snipers to be seen were the ones working on my side, since technically the "enemy" had been removed the day of my lumpectomy, and no stray cancer cells were ever found.

If I may use a political analogy, chemotherapy felt sort of like attacking a country because we thought it was a threat, even though no one turned up any WMD (Weapons of Me Destruction).

Real warriors risk their lives and suffer deprivations far from their homes and loved ones. They return to their families twisted and mangled and psychologically damaged in ways we probably can't imagine unless we personally know, or have been, an injured soldier. Support for them is decidedly uneven—good in some ways, disgracefully inadequate in others. Breast cancer truly sucks, but it does not require of us the kinds of sacrifices that true warriors willingly make every day.

So, if I won't call myself a survivor or a warrior, what should I call myself?

How about a NED? It's an abbreviation for No Evidence of Disease that I discovered on one of the breast cancer message boards. A lot of message posters use it to describe their condition—I think it comes straight off their medical charts. I like the idea—it's factual more than wishful—but it's *Ned*, a name I associate with Ned Flanders, the Simpsons' goofy neighbor.

"Okily dokily, Doctoreeno" just doesn't sound like me.

NED is also an acronym for No Expiration Date, which sounds pretty attractive; I would love to have no expiration date.

But I can't go around saying, "Hi, I'm NED."

And to be perfectly honest, there's another reason words like "survivor" and "warrior" make me uncomfortable. When "breast cancer survivor" becomes the standardized way of describing a person with breast cancer, it allows us to forget about another equally valid description: victim.

254

Nobody likes to use that word, and I don't either, but "victim" is a completely appropriate term sometimes, and a necessary one.

Because not everyone is a survivor. Far too many are victims. By only using the word "survivor" we lull ourselves into a rosy, feel-good complacency, with an incomplete picture of what breast cancer truth really is. Yes, the vast majority of breast cancer patients will live on and be fine, but forty thousand, every year, won't.

Forty thousand women—that's more than thirteen times the number of people killed in the World Trade Center attack. As I write this it happens to be October, and in searching the major breast cancer Web sites for references or memorials to the women who died last year, I find almost nothing. Literally. And that includes the political breast cancer bloggers, the ragers against the Pink Machine.

I did, however, find a Web site that was selling a lovely variety of "In Memory Of____" sweatshirts, T-shirts, and hoodies.

It has been more than twenty-one years since October was designated Breast Cancer Awareness Month. The movement is officially an adult, and I would like it to grow up. It doesn't have to tell only the survivors' stories. We don't need the message to be sugar-coated and wrapped with pink ribbons. We don't have to be assured that breast cancer will make us better people for having gone through it. We don't have to try to convince ourselves that it is a gift, and that if we don't think it is, we're too negative.

We can handle the whole truth about breast cancer. The truth will save lives, in the long run, because it will allow us to understand that, for all the progress made, it remains a terrible, gruesome killer. No amount of teddy bears, bracelets, pink ribbons, or pink angels will change that fact. It will take science and the continued determination of some very tough, politically savvy advocates.

The personal is political, and breast cancer is about as personal as it gets.

I would rather be called "advocate" than "survivor."

What I will advocate is the maturing of the breast cancer movement, untying the pink ribbons that seem to be blinders for so many sincere and dedicated activists. Let us begin to talk about the whole breast cancer picture, what we can do as individuals, what we must do as citizens and consumers to end this epidemic.

Furthermore, the breast cancer community has a special place in the public's consciousness, and I think that gives us a special obligation to speak out on behalf of those who are overlooked and under–cared for. Which in this country is pretty much anybody who doesn't have adequate access to affordable health care, but just to use one example, let's take someone with ovarian cancer.

September is Ovarian Cancer Awareness Month; did you know that? I didn't, either. If ever a disease could benefit from a public awareness campaign, it's ovarian cancer—hard to detect early, and very difficult to cure when detected late. Women who have it realize very few people know about them and what they go through. They don't begrudge breast cancer patients all the support they can muster, but they would very much appreciate more support themselves.

Ovarian cancer is far less common than breast cancer—about twenty-two thousand women will be diagnosed with it this year—but it is also far less curable. More than fifteen thousand women will die of it this year. When it's caught before it's spread outside the ovaries, 90 percent of patients will survive at least five years. But when it's detected after it's spread, the five-year survival rate drops to under 25 percent.

Tragically, the vast majority of cases are detected after it's spread. And yet, the National Cancer Institute will spend about seven times more on breast cancer than on ovarian cancer research. It seems to me that the awesome power of the breast cancer advocacy movement could lend some political muscle to our sisters who desperately need it.

Just Say No to Special Treatment for Breast Cancer?

One way to help might be to insist that instead of singling out breast cancer for certain protections, national policy include everyone who needs protection.

There is a bill before Congress, first introduced in 1997

and reintroduced in 2007, called the Breast Cancer Patient Protection Act. Its goal is to mandate that insurance companies allow mastectomy patients to stay in the hospital for no fewer than two days. Sounds more than reasonable, doesn't it? Lifetime television thinks so; they've had a petition drive on their Web site for years, and they've collected 14 million signatures. Naturally, many of the breast cancer advocacy groups think it's an excellent idea.

But it's not actively supported by the National Breast Cancer Coalition, nor by Breast Cancer Action. Why not? Because, among other reasons, both organizations think it's wrong and unfair to cherry-pick one group, even when it's breast cancer patients, for special protections. Here's how the women at Breast Cancer Action put it:

> *Why should breast cancer patients be any different than all the others with debilitating illnesses who must suffer short hospital stays because of harsh insurance company policies and a generally disastrous health care system? The legislation encourages a trend of piece-meal legislation that wins rights for limited groups one-at-a-time instead of addressing the larger problem of an impersonal managed care system and the lack of universal access to quality health care.*

Yup, that sounds right to me. I've always believed—before, during, and after breast cancer—that our government is supposed to provide for its citizens, not just its corporations, and that every society has to take care of its people to the fullest extent possible, not the minimum amount it can get away with.

Once again I find that breast cancer didn't change me, but it did confirm what's important to me.

As you get back to your life, you're bound to have some new goals, like, say, letting your hair grow to the middle of your back. Or quitting a job you've never enjoyed. I admit I have less patience for work that isn't fulfilling. Mostly, I have the same goals as before, but I'm more eager to try to accomplish them.

I began this book with a quote from Karl Wallenda, the patriarch of the family of tightrope walkers, because what I had begun doing with my life just before the moment I learned I had breast cancer felt like a thrilling but risky high-wire act.

I said that like Wallenda, I would do my act without a safety net. But that was only how I felt at the time, not how it really was. Financially speaking, I did have a safety net—I had enough money to live on for a while, and decent, although not nearly adequate, insurance. I also had the support of a loving family. But equally as important, I had faith that if I did fall, I would be able to find a way to land safely and get back up again.

I'll bet you have a safety net built on your life's experiences, too, even if you've never had to test it before.

The trick is to remember it's there, and to have faith in your own powers when the unexpected happens—when suddenly there's a gust of wind, a missed step, a mistake. Trust in ourselves keeps us moving forward until we've made it all the way across the wire to the safety of the other side.

Oh, and by the way ...

The first time the Wallendas performed at Madison Square Garden without a net, it was only because of a mistake; the net had been lost in shipping. The Wallendas might have been scared, but they clearly had enough faith in their abilities to do their act anyway.

And the reason their name changed from the Great Wallendas to the Flying Wallendas was because of another mistake, an accident—four of them fell out of the pyramid formation they were attempting, but they managed to hold on to the wire. A newspaper reporter said they were so graceful it looked as though they were flying, not falling. Voila, the Flying Wallendas.

I love it when real life is more poetic than a metaphor.

Next time I find myself falling, I'm going to try to remember to fly.

Breast cancer didn't transform me. It didn't reform me. It did sort of deform me, but only a little. It's not so bad.

After an interruption for technical difficulties, I've rejoined my life, already in progress.

About the Author

Shelley Lewis spent nearly thirty years in the broadcast news business, producing radio and television programming at NBC, ABC and CNN. She began at NBC radio, with stints as a features reporter, sports commentator and movie reviewer. For most of her career, she produced television news programs, ranging from *NBC News at Sunrise* and *Real Life with Jane Pauley,* to *ABC's World News Now* and *Good Morning America.* At CNN, she produced a late-night program, an early-morning program, and extensive coverage of 9/11 and the Iraq war. In 2004, she left CNN to help create and launch Air America Radio.

She is cofounder and chief programming executive of the Web site Howdini.com.

In 2006, she published her first book, *Naked Republicans: A Full-Frontal Exposure of Right-Wing Hypocrisy and Greed,* a satirical voter's guide.

A graduate of NYU School of the Arts, she lives in New York with her husband. Their daughter is in college.